IN THE SERIES

The Human Side of Medical Training

Learning Under Pressure

Studying for Medical School

Scrubs and Support

When Things Don't Go As Planned

Before You Decide You're the Problem

How to Make Sense of Struggle, Feedback, and Progress in Medical School

Laura S. Woodward, Ph.D.

THRESHOLD ACADEMIC PRESS

Royal Oak, Michigan

This book is intended for educational purposes only. It does not provide medical or mental health care and is not a substitute for professional care, academic advising, clinical supervision, or institutional guidance. The frameworks and examples presented here are intended to support thinking about learning and performance under pressure, not to diagnose or treat distress.

Readers experiencing persistent or worsening distress, illness, substantial difficulty functioning, concerns about safety, or academic difficulties beyond the scope of this book should seek support appropriate to the situation from qualified professionals, supervisors, advisors, or institutional resources.

The information in this book reflects the author's interpretation of research and educational practice at the time of writing. Research findings, educational practices, and institutional policies may change over time.

The author drew on professional experience, established research, and standard editorial tools in the preparation of this work. Digital tools, including language-assistance technologies, were used selectively to support drafting and editing. All conceptual frameworks, interpretations, and final editorial decisions are the author's own.

First edition.

ISBN: 979-8-9947927-8-0

Library of Congress Control Number: 2026922139

Printed in the United States of America

thresholdacademicpress@gmail.com

Contents

INTRODUCTION

A Difficult Performance Is Not a Diagnosis

You may have entered medical school accustomed to being capable. You may not have felt confident all the time, but you had evidence that you could learn difficult things, work hard, and figure out what was expected of you.

Then the conditions changed. Maybe it was the first anatomy exam that did not go the way you expected, the first OSCE where your mind seemed to empty as soon as someone started watching, or the first morning on the wards when everyone else appeared to know where to stand, what to say, and what mattered.

Sometimes the change is quieter. You had been doing fine, then you started a new block, joined a new team, or took on more responsibility. Something that had begun to feel manageable became difficult again.

You miss a question you thought you knew. Your presentation wanders, you forget something obvious, or someone corrects you in front of the team. Later, when the day has moved on for everyone else, you are still replaying the moment.

Why couldn't I do that? is a reasonable question, and it deserves an answer. *Am I actually bad at this?* sounds like another question, but it already contains a conclusion.

Medical school gives you constant information about your performance, and some of that information matters enormously. The problem is that a difficult performance does not arrive with an explanation attached.

A Finding Is Not a Diagnosis

Imagine that a patient develops shortness of breath. The symptom matters, so you would take it seriously. You would also ask what changed, what else is happening, which explanations fit, and what needs attention now.

Your own difficult moments deserve some of the same discipline. When a performance changes, the change is worth noticing before you decide what caused it.

Suppose a resident asks why your patient's creatinine increased, and you cannot give a coherent answer. One explanation is straightforward: you do not understand the relevant physiology well enough, and you need to learn it.

That possibility matters. A framework that protects you from discovering a real gap would be useless.

Other explanations remain possible. You may understand the physiology but have trouble retrieving it quickly enough. You may retrieve several relevant ideas and struggle to decide which one matters for this patient.

You may know what you want to say but have trouble organizing the answer while the team waits. You may also be on your second morning on the service, trying to answer while following the patient list, remembering who everyone is, and working out what your resident expects you to know without looking anything up.

From the outside, these possibilities can produce the same finding: you did not answer well. From the inside, they can collapse into a much larger conclusion about whether you belong here. That is the distinction I want you to keep throughout this book.

A difficult performance is a finding. What you decide it means is an interpretation. Neither identifies the explanation by itself.

The Developmental Differential

Medical training can make quick interpretations tempting because the stakes feel high. When you care deeply about becoming competent, an ordinary performance problem can acquire meaning far beyond the event itself.

You freeze during a presentation and decide you are bad under pressure. Your attending corrects you several times and you wonder whether you are behind. You watch another student move through the day more easily and decide they have something you do not.

Sometimes those interpretations contain useful information. Sometimes they are larger than the evidence allows.

The difference is difficult to see when you are the person who just had the bad day. A more useful approach is to separate the finding from the interpretation long enough to investigate.

I will call this approach the **Developmental Differential**. The Developmental Differential is practical language for this book, not a validated diagnostic or educational model.

The name borrows a familiar habit from medicine: when one finding has several plausible explanations, you keep them open long enough to gather evidence and see which one deserves the most weight.

The same discipline can help with your own performance. A **possible explanation** is one plausible account of what happened. A **working hypothesis** is the one currently best supported by the evidence you have.

Neither needs to become permanent. Your response gives you more information, and what happens next may strengthen the working hypothesis or force you to revise it.

Many hard moments need a useful next move, not a full investigation. A Deeper Differential becomes useful when a problem repeats, persists, carries higher stakes, or remains difficult to explain.

When you do need it, start with three questions:

- **What changed?**
- **Where did the performance break down?**
- **What does the evidence support doing next?**

Those questions will become more precise as the book progresses. For now, their purpose is to interrupt the jump from *something went badly* to *I know what this means about me.*

Try It on One Bad Moment

Think of one recent moment in medical school that still bothers you. Choose something specific enough that you could describe what happened without first explaining why it happened.

It might be a question you missed, a presentation that went badly, an exam score that surprised you, or a procedure that felt much harder than expected. It could also be one of those days when everyone else seemed to be moving at normal speed while you spent the afternoon trying to catch up.

Take five minutes and write two things:

- **What happened:** Describe what someone watching could reasonably have observed.
- **What I decided it meant:** Write the conclusion you drew about yourself, your ability, or your future.

For example:

- **What happened:** "I could not answer my resident's question about why the patient's sodium was falling."
- **What I decided it meant:** "I am too far into medical school to be missing questions like this."

Notice the distance between those two lines. The interpretation may contain something important. Perhaps you really do need to review the physiology, and discovering that now gives you a specific problem you can address.

The problem may also be different. Perhaps you knew the physiology but could not retrieve it, understood the pieces but could not prioritize them, or had not realized what kind of answer your resident was asking for.

Keep the finding and the interpretation separate for now. Deciding what it means can wait.

Make It Testable

Suppose you decide that a knowledge gap is one possible explanation. The next question is what evidence would make that explanation more or less plausible.

Can you explain the physiology later, when nobody is waiting, or does the explanation remain incomplete even with time to think? Does the same difficulty appear when you work through a similar case?

Those observations change the differential. If you still cannot explain the concept later, a knowledge gap becomes more plausible. If the explanation returns readily once the immediate demands have passed, difficulty accessing what you know becomes more plausible.

Neither observation settles the question by itself. Knowledge and access can fail together, and a later explanation may benefit from time, cues, or reconstruction. The point is narrower: the next performance gives you better evidence about where to look.

You still may not know exactly what happened after one event. That is fine. A working hypothesis only needs to be good enough to guide a useful next step.

You might review the concept, practice retrieving it from a clinical prompt, ask what kind of answer your resident expected, or watch what happens the next time a similar question arises. The response becomes part of the investigation because the result gives you new evidence.

This is the rhythm the rest of the book will use:

1. **finding**
2. **interpretation**
3. **possible explanations**
4. **working hypothesis**
5. **response**
6. **reassessment**

Evidence runs through the entire process. It helps you decide which explanation deserves attention now and whether that explanation still fits after you act.

The Questions Get More Specific

The rest of this book will make the investigation more precise. You will ask what changed around you, where the performance actually broke down, and whether the task itself changed as you advanced.

You will also examine the evidence you are using to judge yourself. A feeling, a supervisor's comment, another student's performance, and a repeated pattern across several settings do not necessarily support the same conclusions.

Later, the social conditions of learning enter the investigation more explicitly. You will look at role, hierarchy, help-seeking, uncertainty, capacity, and what happens when part of your attention leaves the work and begins watching you do the work.

These are different problems, but the method underneath them stays recognizable:

Describe what happened. Distinguish among plausible explanations. Choose a response that fits the evidence. See what happens next.

Memorizing a collection of frameworks won't help. What you need is a way to think when the alternative is a global conclusion such as *I am getting worse* or *I am not cut out for this.*

What the Differential Cannot Do

There is an important boundary around this framework. A developmental explanation should never become a convenient way to explain away a pattern that needs attention.

If you repeatedly struggle with the same important task after expectations are clear and you have had appropriate opportunities to learn and practice, let that pattern matter. If several people who have observed your work are giving you similar feedback, that convergence deserves attention too.

The same is true when the problem is larger than ordinary learning difficulty. Any of the following requires support or intervention appropriate to the situation:

- Persistent impairment
- Unsafe performance
- Severe distress
- Illness
- Inadequate supervision
- Mistreatment
- Discrimination
- Another harmful condition

The Developmental Differential cannot tell you that every difficult experience is normal. It can help you determine what kind of problem you may be dealing with before you choose a response.

Sometimes the answer may point to something that needs real attention. You may need:

- more knowledge
- more practice
- direct feedback
- closer supervision
- help with something affecting your ability to function

Sometimes the environment will be part of the explanation. Your responsibility to learn does not make every expectation reasonable, every supervision arrangement adequate, or every training environment safe.

Accuracy matters in both directions. A correctable knowledge gap deserves to be identified accurately, and so does a problem created or intensified by the conditions under which you are being asked to learn.

Before You Decide

Medical school can give you many opportunities to feel incompetent, and some of those moments will expose things you genuinely need to learn. Others will happen because you are trying to use what you know under conditions that changed before you had time to become familiar with them.

Later, the task may change too. You may be asked to prioritize instead of list, decide instead of report, act with less prompting, and recognize when you need help.

Often, several explanations will be true at once. That is why the purpose of this book is not to convince you that you are doing better than you think.

The goal is to help you become more accurate about what difficult moments mean. Accuracy gives you a better chance of choosing a response that fits the problem.

A knowledge gap can lead to targeted study. A retrieval problem may call for practice bringing the knowledge forward when it is needed.

An unclear expectation can be clarified. An unreliable skill can be practiced with observation and feedback.

A supervision problem requires a different response. A harmful condition may need to be named and brought to people with the authority or expertise to help.

A global judgment such as *I'm just bad at this* gives you far less to work with. It collapses different problems into one conclusion and then asks you to improve yourself in general.

So when something becomes harder, try not to settle its meaning before you have investigated the event. Describe what happened, keep plausible explanations open, and gather enough evidence to decide what deserves your attention next.

You may still discover a problem that needs work. The difference is that you will have something more useful than a verdict about yourself. You will have a working hypothesis, a next move, and a way to find out whether you were right.

This book is about ordinary developmental difficulty — performance that changes as the task, environment, or expectations around you change. If a specific event brought you here instead — a failed exam, a remediation notice, a formal setback that now needs a recovery plan — *When Things Don't Go As Planned* stays with that event and what comes next.

A NOTE BEFORE YOU BEGIN

How to Use This Book

You do not have to use every framework in this book, underline every sentence, or complete every reflection. This is not meant to turn your already crowded life into another improvement project. It is meant to help you pause long enough to ask a better question: *What changed?*

Most chapters can be read one at a time. You can come to the chapter that matches the transition you are in, the kind of difficulty you are having, or the sentence you keep repeating to yourself. You can leave the rest for later.

When your bandwidth is low, start with the Recap, the Stabilizing Shift, or the simplest question in the chapter. Sometimes the most useful move is not a full analysis. It is noticing one change in the task, one missing piece of feedback, one unclear expectation, or one place where a strategy that used to work no longer fits the situation you are in.

Use the smallest version of this that helps. You do not need to investigate yourself endlessly.

This matters because reflection can help, but it can also become rumination. If a tool in this book helps you understand the situation more clearly, use it. If it makes you circle the same fear again and again, put it down. The goal is not to prove that everything is fine. The goal is to understand the problem well enough to choose the next useful support, strategy, conversation, or correction.

There are also times when this book is not enough. If the problem involves safety, severe distress, impaired functioning, mistreatment, discrimination, unsafe supervision, illness, formal academic action, or concern that you may harm yourself or someone else, do not try to solve it only by reflecting harder. Use appropriate institutional, professional, clinical, crisis, disability, reporting, advising, or supervisory support.

This book can help you interpret difficulty. It should not become a reason to stay alone with something that needs more help than a book can provide.

This book is about interpreting difficulty before it becomes a verdict. It does not replace a study system, a remediation plan, mental health care, academic advising, clinical supervision, disability support, reporting pathways, or institutional help. It helps you ask better questions before choosing which of those supports or strategies may fit.

A one-page version of this map — the same questions, none of the elaboration — is waiting at the back of the book whenever you want it.

Note for Someone Reading Alongside a Trainee

If someone who loves you is reading this with you, the purpose is not to help them diagnose what is wrong. It is to help both of you slow down the leap from difficulty to verdict.

The best support often sounds less like, *You're fine,* and more like, *Let's understand what changed before we decide what this means.*

If the problem is mainly how someone close to you can support a medical trainee without adding pressure, *Scrubs and Support* goes further. This book stays focused on the learner's experience of transition, interpretation, and adaptation.

A Few Places to Look Next

If the problem is mainly study design, scheduling, retention, or exam preparation, *Studying for Medical School* goes further.

If the problem is mainly what happens when a plan falls apart, a course does not go as expected, or a setback requires repair, *When Things Don't Go As Planned* may be the better companion.

If someone close to you is trying to help without increasing pressure, *Scrubs and Support* may be useful.

You do not need all of them at once. Use the book that matches the problem in front of you.

PART I

When Something Suddenly Gets Harder

You were getting better at this, and then something changed. A task that had started to feel manageable suddenly requires more thought, effort, or attention than it did before.

The new block starts, and routines that worked last week no longer work quite as smoothly. You know how to present a patient, but this team wants the presentation organized differently. Or you studied the material but cannot use it as quickly as you expected when someone asks you a clinical question.

Later in training, the experience can become even more confusing. You know more than you used to know, yet the work may feel harder when you are given less prompting, asked to make more decisions, or expected to recognize what matters before someone tells you.

These situations can produce the same conclusion: *I was getting better. Why do I suddenly feel worse?* Part I separates three questions that can help make that experience more specific.

What Changed Around Me?

Start with the widest view. Before deciding that something changed in you, ask whether the conditions surrounding the performance changed.

A new block can change the people, workflow, expectations, supervision, responsibility, and unwritten rules surrounding a task. Familiar work may therefore become less fluent even when much of what you already know is still available to you.

Chapter 1 will help you identify those changes without assuming that the environment explains every difficulty. Sometimes the new setting is part of the explanation. Sometimes it reveals a gap that was already there.

Where Did the Performance Break Down?

If the environment does not explain enough, move closer to the performance itself. Ask where the difficulty actually occurred instead of treating the visible result as its own explanation.

You may lack knowledge you need, or you may know the material and have trouble accessing it when the situation requires it. You may retrieve the relevant information but struggle to decide what matters most, or you may know what you want to do and have difficulty executing it reliably.

The environment can also interfere with performance through unclear expectations, interruptions, workflow, or inadequate support. Chapter 2 will help you distinguish among **Knowledge, Access, Prioritization, Execution, and Environment** so that the response can fit the point where the performance actually broke down.

Did the Task Itself Change?

Sometimes the environment is becoming familiar and the underlying knowledge is growing, yet the work still becomes harder. In that situation, ask whether the task carrying the familiar name is actually asking something new of you.

You may still be told to *present the patient*, while the expected performance has shifted from reporting information toward selecting what matters. You may still be asked to develop a plan, while the work now requires integrating competing information, committing to a judgment, or recognizing when your usual approach no longer fits.

A familiar task can therefore become more demanding without being renamed. Chapter 3 asks how to recognize when the work underneath the label has changed—and how to test that explanation rather than assume it.

Three Questions Before a Verdict

Part I moves through three progressively narrower questions:

- **What changed around me?**
- **Where did the performance break down?**
- **Did the task itself change?**

You will not need all three every time something goes badly. The point is not to perform a complete analysis after every difficult day.

Often, one question will make the problem specific enough to choose a useful next move. You may need to learn the new environment, work on the point where the performance broke down, or identify what the current version of the task requires.

The investigation may reveal a genuine gap in knowledge or skill. It may reveal that several explanations are operating together. Or it may show that the task you thought you were failing is no longer quite the task you first learned to do.

Part I begins with the widest view because context is easy to miss when the performance feels personal. **Before you decide that you changed, look carefully at what changed around you.**

CHAPTER ONE

Why a New Block Can Make You Feel New Again

By 7:12 a.m., you are already behind.

You found the team room after checking two hallways and asking someone at the nurses' station. You know which patients are yours, but you are still figuring out where this service keeps the information you need and which parts of the chart your resident expects you to review before rounds.

You start presenting your first patient. Thirty seconds in, your attending interrupts and asks for the overnight events before the rest of the history. You adjust, then spend the next two presentations trying to remember whether this attending wants the assessment before or after the new data.

None of this is especially dramatic. By noon, it can still leave you feeling strangely incompetent.

Last Friday, you knew what you were doing. On Monday, ordinary tasks require concentration again.

The tempting explanation is that you somehow lost ground over the weekend. A more useful first question is simpler: **What changed around you?**

If you are not yet in clinical rotations, the same question may show up after a quiz, anatomy practical, small-group case, simulation, lab, standardized patient encounter, or the first time you realize that knowing the material and using it under pressure are not the same experience. The transition may be smaller, but the interpretive risk is similar: a changed task can feel like a changed self.

You Did Not Start Over

A new block changes more than the patients you see. It can change the people, workflow, schedule, physical space, documentation habits, expectations, supervision, resources, and routines surrounding the work.

Research on the transition into clinical training describes it as more than a change of setting. Students are entering a different educational and social environment, forming new relationships, learning unfamiliar norms, and finding ways to participate in clinical work (Atherley et al., 2019; Teunissen & Westerman, 2011). Workplace-learning research similarly emphasizes participation in clinical practice as central to how medical students learn in clinical settings (Dornan et al., 2007).

That distinction matters because much of what made you efficient last week may have depended on familiarity with the environment. You knew where to find information, which tasks happened first, what your supervisor cared about, whom to ask, and which details could safely wait.

Once those routines become familiar, you no longer have to think as deliberately about each one. When the environment changes, many become questions again.

The resulting difficulty can feel surprisingly global. *I don't know how to do this* may be the thought that arrives even when a more precise description is *I don't yet know how this place does this.*

That difference is the starting point for Chapter 1. A change in fluency does not establish a loss of competence.

Some Competence Travels. Some Fluency Is Local.

Changing rotations did not erase what you already learned. Some of your competence travels with you — knowledge, skills, judgment, and clinical habits carried from one setting into another, even when you cannot yet use all of it with the same ease.

Some fluency is more local. The ease you developed in one setting may depend partly on routines, relationships, expectations, and conditions specific to that setting. I use local fluency here as descriptive language for that context-dependent ease, not as a validated construct.

Last week, you knew where the patient list lived, when to start prerounding, how much detail your resident wanted, and which information your attending expected you to have ready. You may barely have noticed that knowledge because you no longer had to work hard to use it.

Then the block changed. Suddenly you are asking questions that have little to do with whether you understand medicine:

- *Where do I meet the team?*
- *What does "prerounded" mean here?*
- *How detailed should this presentation be?*
- *Which results am I expected to follow myself?*
- *When should I tell my resident about a change?*
- *What can I do independently?*

These questions are part of learning how to function in a clinical workplace. They also require attention while you are trying to do the medicine.

This is why the first days of a new block can feel harder than your knowledge alone would predict. You may be bringing substantial competence into an environment where you have very little local fluency.

The Work Around the Work

Consider what it takes to present one patient on the first morning of a new service. You need to understand the patient. You may also need to locate the chart, learn where overnight events are documented, determine which laboratory results matter to this team, find your resident, remember the order of rounds, infer how much detail the attending wants, and work out which parts of the plan you are expected to propose yourself.

The presentation is the visible task. Around it sits another layer of activity required to make the presentation possible.

I will call this **the work around the work**. The phrase is descriptive rather than another framework you need to remember.

In a familiar environment, much of this surrounding work can fade into the background. When the environment changes, it becomes visible again: you are locating, remembering, inferring, deciding, and doing things that recently required less deliberate thought.

That gives you a useful observational question when a familiar task suddenly feels difficult: **What am I trying to locate, remember, infer, decide, and do simultaneously?**

The question does not tell you why the task is harder. It helps you see what else the task currently requires.

Suppose your presentation is slower on Monday than it was on Friday. If Monday also requires you to navigate a new chart workflow, infer a new presentation standard, remember new team roles, and decide what you are responsible for following, the slower presentation now has context.

That context does not prove that the environment caused the problem. It does tell you that *my presentations are getting worse* is too early a conclusion.

The Rotation Reset

This recurring experience is useful to name. I will call it the **Rotation Reset**.

A Rotation Reset is a reduction in local fluency that can occur when you enter a new learning environment — a drop in the routines that let you use what you already know efficiently. The term is explanatory language for this book, not a validated educational construct. Its purpose is to help you recognize a recurring pattern without turning that pattern into a diagnosis.

You may notice a Rotation Reset when a new clerkship begins, when you change hospitals or teams, or when you move from one kind of clinical work to another. A similar experience can occur when you return after an extended period away.

Imagine returning to a hospital after leave. The building is familiar, and you recognize the electronic record, but routines that once happened automatically now require deliberate thought.

You pause to remember where to find a result, which screen you used to review medications, or how you organized your morning before rounds. That experience does not tell us that leave necessarily produced a deficit, and it does not tell us why any particular learner is struggling. It illustrates a narrower point: local fluency can need rebuilding even when the environment itself is technically familiar.

Clarify What Matters Early

Once you recognize that some of the difficulty is local, the next move is not to learn every preference and unwritten rule immediately. Many can become clearer as you participate in the work.

Prioritize expectations that affect safe participation and your ability to contribute appropriately: what you are responsible for, which decisions require supervision, what information needs to be communicated promptly, and what your supervisor considers a useful performance of the task. A few bounded questions can reduce unnecessary guessing:

- "What should I make sure I know before rounds?"
- "What does a strong presentation look like to you?"
- "Which decisions should I make myself, and which should I run by you?"
- "What changes do you want me to tell you about right away?"

You do not need to conduct an interview with every new supervisor. Ask the questions whose answers will change what you do.

Other local rules can emerge as you work. Chapter 6 will return to what happens when important expectations remain invisible, and Chapter 8 will address what happens when asking appropriate questions or seeking help carries social costs. For now, the principle is smaller: clarify consequential expectations early enough that you are not trying to infer everything while also performing.

Watch What Familiarity Changes

A Rotation Reset becomes useful as an explanation only if it gives you something to watch. Think back to the first morning. You had to find the team, work out where information lived, learn the sequence of the morning, and infer what your supervisor wanted.

Three days later, some of those questions may require less effort. You know where to meet, where to find the relevant information, and roughly how rounds work.

A week later, you may be spending less attention on navigation and more on the patients themselves. Your presentation may become more concise because you understand which details matter to this team.

That trajectory gives you evidence. **If the difficulty decreases as the environment becomes familiar, that pattern supports local fluency as part of the original explanation.**

Notice what this does not tell you. It does not prove that every problem was caused by the transition, and it does not tell you that any remaining difficulty should be ignored.

It gives you a prediction. If unfamiliarity is contributing substantially, some parts of the work should become easier as familiarity grows.

If It Does Not Improve, Reopen the Differential

Now imagine that the workflow becomes familiar, but your presentations remain disorganized. You know where to find the information and what your attending expects, yet you still struggle to identify which findings matter enough to emphasize.

The Rotation Reset no longer explains enough. Something else deserves investigation.

Perhaps you need more knowledge to understand which findings are clinically important. Perhaps the knowledge is there, but prioritization remains difficult.

Maybe you can organize the case on paper but struggle to do it aloud. That would point toward a different part of the performance.

This is why transition is not an indefinite explanation. An explanation that fit the first few days needs revision when the trajectory stops supporting it.

The same rule protects against the opposite error. If you struggle on the first morning of every new rotation and reliably become more fluent once you understand the environment, repeatedly treating those first mornings as evidence of declining ability ignores your own trajectory.

Watch what changes with familiarity. Then let the evidence update the explanation.

What to Do in the First Forty-Eight Hours

You do not need to master a new environment immediately. Aim for enough orientation to reduce avoidable uncertainty and enough observation to see what becomes easier with exposure.

During the first day or two, identify the basic workflow and the expectations that affect safety, responsibility, and your ability to contribute. Ask where you need to be, what you are responsible for knowing or following, what requires supervision, and what a useful version of your core task looks like.

Then pay attention to what stops requiring so much thought. Notice which routines become automatic, which expectations become clearer, and which difficulties remain even after the surrounding work becomes easier.

In the first forty-eight hours, you are gathering evidence about what belongs to the transition and what may require a different response. You do not need to explain your entire performance during those first days. You need enough information to know what to learn about the environment and what to keep watching.

Before You Decide You Got Worse

A new block can make a capable student feel unexpectedly new. The medicine may be familiar while the conditions for using it have changed.

Some competence travels with you, while some fluency depends partly on a particular place, team, workflow, or routine. When that local fluency drops, the work around the work becomes visible again.

That is the Rotation Reset. Recognizing it gives you a hypothesis, not a complete explanation.

Clarify the expectations that matter, learn the local workflow, and watch what improves as the environment becomes familiar. If the difficulty improves with familiarity, you have learned something about what changed.

If it persists, return to the differential with more information. The next question is no longer simply *What changed around me?*

It becomes more precise: **Where did the performance actually break down?**

Stabilizing Shift

When a familiar task suddenly feels harder, ask what changed around you before you ask what changed in you.

Naming that shift the Rotation Reset gives you a hypothesis to test, not a verdict to accept.

Options Menu

- **Ask a bounded question.** Try "What should I make sure I know before rounds?" or "What does a strong presentation look like to you?" — pick the ones whose answers will actually change what you do.
- **Watch the trajectory.** Give the new environment a few days and notice what becomes easier. That pattern is evidence, not just a feeling.
- **Name the Rotation Reset.** If the drop in fluency fits the pattern — new team, new workflow, same underlying competence — treat it as the working explanation for now.
- **Reopen the differential.** If your presentations stay disorganized after the workflow becomes familiar, look at Chapter 2's Knowledge, Access, Prioritization, Execution, and Environment categories instead.

Common Trap

Comparing this week's performance to last week's, as though the test stayed the same. That comparison protects a felt sense of continuity, but it treats a new team, workflow, and set of expectations as if they were unchanged.

A calmer alternative: withhold the comparison until you have had a few days in the new environment, then check whether the gap is closing.

Recap

What to remember when stressed:

- A new block can make old competence feel unreliable — that is not the same as losing it.
- Some competence travels with you; some fluency is local to a place, team, or routine.
- Clarify a few consequential expectations early, rather than guessing at all of them.
- Watch what improves as the environment becomes familiar — that trajectory is evidence.
- If the difficulty does not improve, reopen the differential in Chapter 2.

CHAPTER TWO

You Knew This Yesterday. Why Can't You Do It Today?

Yesterday, you knew this.

You could explain the physiology while studying, recognize the diagnosis in a question bank, and tell a classmate why one answer made more sense than the others. Then your resident asks you about the same concept on rounds, and your mind goes blank.

Or the information does come back, but too much of it arrives at once. You can name six things that might explain the patient's new anemia, but when your attending asks which one you think is most likely, you cannot decide what matters most.

Sometimes you know exactly what you want to do and still cannot do it reliably. Your patient presentation has a clear structure when you rehearse it, then becomes disorganized once you are standing in front of the team.

These experiences can produce the same conclusion: *I need to study more.* Sometimes that conclusion is correct, while sometimes the problem was never primarily about missing information.

That distinction matters because the same bad performance can come from different problems. **Different problems need different responses.**

This does not begin only when you enter the hospital. In the preclinical years, you may notice it when the study method that worked for one block stops working in the next, when a familiar lecture format becomes an application-heavy exam, or when a standardized patient encounter asks you to integrate knowledge, presence, language, and timing all at once. Before deciding that you have lost your ability, ask whether the task has become more integrated than the strategy you are using.

Start With Where the Performance Broke Down

Suppose you cannot answer a question about why a patient's sodium is falling. The visible problem is straightforward: you did not answer the question well.

That finding does not tell you where the performance broke down. You may never have understood the relevant physiology, or you may understand it and have trouble retrieving it without cues.

You may retrieve several relevant ideas but struggle to identify which one fits this patient. You may know what you think and have difficulty expressing the reasoning clearly enough for someone else to follow.

Something in the environment may also have interfered with the performance. You may have been interrupted, working under unfamiliar conditions, or trying to complete several competing tasks when the question arrived.

For this book, it helps to separate five places where performance can break down:

- **Knowledge**
- **Access**
- **Prioritization**
- **Execution**
- **Environment**

These are practical distinctions for investigating a difficult performance, not an established assessment model. They are not claims that every performance failure fits neatly into one box. Several may contribute to the same event.

Their value is simple. Before deciding what to do about a difficult performance, identify which part of the performance most needs attention.

Knowledge: Do I Actually Understand This?

Start with the possibility that the knowledge itself is incomplete. Sometimes you do not know enough yet.

A knowledge problem exists when the information, concept, or relationship you need is missing, incomplete, or insufficiently understood for the task. You may recognize the topic without being able to explain it, or remember isolated facts without understanding how they fit together.

Imagine that your resident asks why a patient with heart failure might develop hyponatremia. Later, with your notes open and nobody waiting, you still cannot explain the physiology coherently.

That is useful information. The problem appears to involve more than performing under pressure because the underlying understanding itself needs work.

The response should match that problem. Return to the relevant material, identify what you do not understand, and build enough understanding that you can explain and use it without leaning continuously on the source.

If Knowledge was the main problem, better understanding should change what you can explain and apply when you encounter the concept again. If it does not, reopen the differential — more studying may have improved your knowledge without solving the part of the performance that originally failed.

Access: Can I Bring Forward What I Know When This Task Requires It?

Now imagine a different version of the same event. You cannot answer on rounds, but twenty minutes later, before you have looked anything up, the explanation returns.

That does not prove that your knowledge was intact. It does tell you something important: what you could produce changed when the conditions changed.

For this book, I will call that an **Access** question: **Can I bring relevant knowledge forward when this task requires it?**

Access is practical language for locating the difficulty, not a separate memory system or a diagnosis. The useful distinction is between needing to build more understanding and needing to become more reliable at producing what you have learned under the conditions in which you will use it.

Knowing information under one set of conditions does not guarantee that you will retrieve it when another task requires it. Retrieval practice can strengthen later retention, and some experimental evidence suggests that its benefits can extend to new questions, although transfer depends on what was practiced and what the later task requires (Roediger & Karpicke, 2006; Butler, 2010; Larsen et al., 2008).

The practical implication can stay modest. If you need to produce knowledge in response to clinical prompts, include practice that requires you to produce it from a clinical prompt.

Close the notes and explain why the sodium is falling. Look at the patient problem and generate the mechanism before checking the answer, or ask yourself what you would say if your resident asked the question now.

Then test the explanation. If Access was the main problem, repeated attempts to bring the knowledge forward without relying on recognition should give you more information about whether retrieval is becoming more reliable.

If you still cannot explain the concept even with time and repeated attempts, move Knowledge back up the differential. The point is to let the next performance distinguish between explanations.

Prioritization: Do I Know Too Much to Know What Matters?

Sometimes retrieval works perfectly well. The problem begins after the information arrives.

Your attending asks why the patient's blood pressure has fallen, and you can generate several plausible explanations. You know the medications, vital signs, laboratory results, overnight events, and relevant physiology.

Then comes the harder question: Which of those things matters most here? Clinical reasoning depends heavily on what a learner knows and how that knowledge is organized for use in particular clinical problems. Research on expertise describes changes in the organization and representation of clinical knowledge with experience rather than a single general reasoning ability (Norman, 2005; Schmidt & Rikers, 2007).

In practice, one place that difference becomes visible is deciding which of several relevant findings deserves the most weight. A prioritization problem can therefore look like a knowledge problem from the outside. The answer is incomplete or unfocused, so the learner concludes that more information must be missing.

More information may not solve the problem if the difficulty lies in deciding which information deserves weight. Suppose your presentation includes every laboratory value, medication change, and overnight event, but your resident repeatedly asks, "What actually matters today?" You may not need another hour of chart review.

You may need help seeing how a more experienced clinician organizes the case. Ask someone to show you which findings they would put first and why, then compare their organization with your own.

If Prioritization was the main problem, clearer guidance about discriminating features and repeated practice deciding what matters should make your reasoning more focused, even without a large increase in factual knowledge. If you still cannot identify the important information because you do not understand what the findings mean, Knowledge returns to the differential.

Execution: Do I Know What to Do but Struggle to Do It Reliably?

You may understand the material, retrieve it, and know what matters. The breakdown can still occur when you try to perform the task.

Perhaps you can describe exactly how you want to present the patient, but your presentation becomes disorganized in real time. You know the steps of a clinical skill but cannot yet carry them out smoothly and reliably.

An execution problem appears when you understand the target but cannot yet produce the performance reliably. In that situation, the next source of information is the performance itself.

Practice the presentation aloud, perform the skill with appropriate supervision, or repeat the relevant sequence while someone observes the part that keeps breaking down. Make the target specific. "Get better at presentations" gives you little to work with, while "state the assessment before adding supporting detail" gives you something observable.

Repeated practice with feedback is well established in some areas of clinical skill acquisition, particularly simulation-based training, although that evidence should not be generalized automatically from one kind of skill to another (McGaghie et al., 2011).

If Execution was the main problem, repeated practice with feedback on the specific performance should make it more reliable. If practice does not help, ask why — you may discover that you were practicing an execution problem while an unresolved Knowledge or Prioritization problem was still underneath it.

Environment: What Changed Around the Performance?

Chapter 1 began with the environment because context can change how difficult a familiar task becomes. The same question belongs here when you investigate a specific performance failure.

Perhaps you normally organize your presentation during chart review, but today you were interrupted repeatedly. Maybe you knew what you wanted to say until a new workflow forced you to switch between several sources of information while trying to keep track of unfinished tasks.

Interruptions are common in clinical work and can affect how tasks unfold or whether they are completed, although their effects depend on the task and setting. The broader evidence does not support treating every interruption as a direct cause of error or harm (Westbrook et al., 2010; Sanderson et al., 2019).

For the learner, begin closer to the event: **What became harder or less reliable after the interruption?**

Then compare. Does the same problem occur when those conditions are absent, or does the performance change substantially when the environment changes?

If Environment is contributing, changing the relevant condition—when possible—may change part of the performance. If the difficulty persists under different conditions, Environment becomes a less complete explanation.

This category also needs a guardrail. Context can also become too complete an explanation.

An interruption may have made the task harder while a knowledge gap still contributed to the mistake. An unfamiliar environment can increase the work around the work while you still need more practice.

The purpose of including Environment is accuracy. It should remain in the differential when the evidence supports it and lose weight when the evidence does not.

A Step 1 Problem That Looks Like "Study More"

The same distinctions apply outside the clinical environment. Imagine that you complete a set of Step 1 practice questions and perform much worse than you expected.

You look at the score and immediately decide that you need three more hours of content review tonight. Pause before assigning the homework. Ask where the performance actually broke down.

If you cannot explain the tested material without your notes, Knowledge is a plausible problem. More focused learning may be appropriate because the underlying understanding is incomplete.

If you recognize the correct explanation immediately when you see it but cannot generate it independently, Access deserves attention. Practice that requires retrieval may be more useful than another pass through material you already recognize.

If you know many facts about the disease but repeatedly miss the clue that distinguishes it from the alternatives, look at Prioritization. The problem may be identifying which feature of the question should change your judgment.

If you know what the question is testing and can solve similar items when untimed but repeatedly run out of time or fail to carry out your approach reliably, examine Execution. You may need to practice the process under conditions closer to the actual task.

If the performance occurred after severe fatigue, repeated interruptions, or unusual testing conditions, Environment belongs in the differential. That does not automatically explain the score, but it gives you a variable to compare against later performances.

The score alone cannot tell you which explanation is correct. **Do not ask three hours of studying to solve a problem that was never primarily about missing information.**

Why Studying More Is Such an Attractive Answer

Studying has several advantages as a response to difficulty. It is familiar, available, measurable, and usually under your control.

It also feels responsible. When something goes badly, opening a textbook or question bank gives you an immediate way to act.

Sometimes that response is well matched. If the problem is Knowledge, targeted study may address the part of the performance that failed.

The trouble begins when studying becomes the default response to every kind of performance problem. You can accumulate more information while leaving the actual breakdown untouched.

If the problem is Access, you may need to retrieve what you already know. If it is Prioritization, you may need help deciding what matters.

If it is Execution, you need to perform the task. If the Environment is interfering, the relevant condition may need clarification, modification, support, or simply recognition as part of the explanation.

The question is therefore more precise than *Should I study more?* Ask: **What would more studying change, and is that the part of the performance that failed?**

Turn the Explanation Into a Prediction

This is the step that keeps the performance differential from becoming a collection of plausible stories. Once you have an explanation, ask: **What would I expect to see if this explanation were right?**

- If you think the problem is Knowledge, what would you expect to improve after targeted study?
- If you think it is Access, what would you expect to change after repeated attempts to retrieve the information without relying on recognition?
- If you think the problem is Prioritization, what might change after someone helps you identify the discriminating information?
- If you think it is Execution, what might become more reliable after focused practice and feedback?
- If you think Environment is contributing, what might change when the relevant condition changes?

Each explanation should make some prediction about the next performance. Then look.

Improvement does not prove that your explanation was completely correct, and lack of improvement does not automatically prove that it was wrong. Human performance is too variable for one attempt to settle every question.

The next performance still gives you evidence. It can strengthen the working hypothesis, weaken it, or show you that several problems were operating together.

That is what keeps the method testable. A useful explanation tells you what to try and what to watch afterward.

Find the Problem You Can Work On

After a difficult performance, you do not need to diagnose yourself perfectly. You need an explanation specific enough to choose a useful next action.

Start with the finding. Describe what actually happened before deciding why it happened.

Then ask where the performance broke down. Did you lack the knowledge, struggle to access it, have difficulty prioritizing what mattered, fail to execute something you understood, or perform under conditions that changed the task?

Choose the explanation that currently has the strongest support and match the response to it. Then ask what you would expect to change if you were right.

Sometimes the answer will be study. Sometimes it will be retrieval practice, help with prioritization, coached performance, or a change in the conditions surrounding the work.

Several explanations may remain plausible, and several may be true. You can still choose the next response that gives you the most useful information.

The visible failure is the beginning of the investigation, not the end of it. **The same bad performance can come from different problems, and different problems need different responses.**

Once you know where the performance broke down, another question becomes possible. Sometimes nothing broke down in the way you first thought. Sometimes the task itself changed.

Stabilizing Shift

Before deciding you need to study more, ask where the performance actually broke down: Knowledge, Access, Prioritization, Execution, or Environment.

The right response depends on which one it was.

Options Menu

- **Test for Knowledge.** Return to the material, then check whether you can explain and apply it — not just recognize it.
- **Test for Access.** Close your notes and try to produce the answer under the same conditions you will actually need it.
- **Test for Prioritization.** Ask someone more experienced which finding they would put first, and why.
- **Test for Execution.** Practice the specific skill aloud or under supervision, rather than reviewing the material again.
- **Test for Environment.** Change the one condition you suspect is interfering, then see whether the same problem still occurs.

Common Trap

Treating every difficult performance as a reason to study more. Studying feels responsible and stays fully within your control, so it can become the default response even when the problem is retrieval, prioritization, execution, or the conditions you were working under.

A calmer alternative: ask what would actually change if you studied more. If nothing in your answer changes, the problem probably is not Knowledge.

Recap

What to remember when stressed:

- The same bad performance can come from different problems: Knowledge, Access, Prioritization, Execution, or Environment.
- Match your response to which one it actually was.
- Turn your explanation into a prediction, then test it on the next performance.
- Studying more only helps if the problem was Knowledge.

- Find the one problem you can work on now — you do not need to diagnose everything at once.

CHAPTER THREE

When the Task Changes but the Name Doesn't

You have done this before. That is part of what makes the difficulty so confusing.

You have studied for exams, presented patients, and completed tasks on a clinical team. Then someone asks you to do what sounds like the same thing, and suddenly your usual approach is not enough.

The assignment still says *study the material*, but recognizing the right answer may no longer be enough. The instruction is still *present the patient*, but listing what happened may no longer be enough.

You are still expected to take care of your patients, but now someone expects you to notice what needs doing before you are prompted. The label stayed the same while the work underneath it changed.

When that happens, the first conclusion may be that you are getting worse. Before you decide that, ask a different question: **Am I actually being asked to do the same task I was doing before?**

For students earlier in training, feedback may arrive as a grade, a missed question pattern, a facilitator's comment, a simulation debrief, or a vague sense that everyone else understood the case faster. These are not all the same kind of evidence. A score may show an outcome without showing the breakdown. A comment may identify a useful pattern, or it may reflect one observer's preference. Part of the work is learning not only from feedback, but how to interpret what kind of feedback you actually received.

The Task Can Change Without Being Renamed

At one point in training, success may depend on doing something relatively easy to name: learn this material, gather this information, complete these steps, or report what you found. Later, an activity with the same name may require additional judgment. You may need to retrieve without cues, distinguish relevant information from noise, compress what you know, commit to an interpretation, or recognize when the familiar approach no longer fits.

The task still has the same name. That continuity can hide how much competent performance now requires.

This matters because you may compare your current effort with an earlier version of the task. *I used to be good at presentations* sounds concerning until you notice that the presentation you are being asked to give now requires more than the one you first learned.

You did not necessarily lose the earlier skill. You may be trying to use it inside a more demanding version of the task.

Sometimes what looks like deteriorating performance may reflect a change in what competent performance now requires. Treat that as a hypothesis to test, not an explanation that advancement automatically supplies.

Studying: From Recognition to Use

Consider studying. Early in a course, you may spend substantial time learning vocabulary, mechanisms, structures, or disease patterns that are genuinely new.

Recognition can initially feel like progress. You see a term or answer choice and know that you have encountered it before.

Later assessments may ask something different. You may need to produce the information without seeing the answer first, distinguish between plausible alternatives, or apply what you know to a problem that does not look exactly like the example you studied.

Imagine that you have reviewed nephrotic and nephritic syndromes several times. You can recognize the characteristic findings when they appear in a table, and you feel reasonably comfortable with the material.

Then a question gives you a patient with edema, hypertension, hematuria, and several additional findings. The task is no longer simply to recognize facts you learned.

You have to retrieve relevant knowledge, decide which findings discriminate among plausible explanations, and apply that knowledge to this particular problem. If you continue studying mainly by rereading the table, you may become increasingly fluent with an earlier version of the task while still struggling with the one you now need to perform.

The point is not that learning always progresses through recognition, retrieval, discrimination, and application in that order. It is that the activity called *studying* can prepare you well for one demand while the assessment requires another.

That changes what you investigate after a disappointing result. Before deciding that you suddenly know less, ask whether the task moved from recognition toward retrieval, discrimination, or application.

If it did, your next practice can give you information about that newer demand. The question becomes whether you can use the knowledge in the way the current task requires.

Presenting: From Reporting to Recommending

The same change can happen in clinical work. When you first learn to present a patient, simply remembering the structure may require substantial effort.

You gather the history, examination findings, laboratory results, imaging, and overnight events. Success may initially mean getting the relevant information into the presentation in a recognizable order.

Then the expectation changes. Your supervisor may no longer need evidence that you can recite everything you found.

Now you may be expected to decide what matters. You need to select information, compress it, interpret it, and make the listener understand what you think is happening.

Eventually, the presentation may need to end somewhere even more demanding: **What do you recommend we do?**

The activity is still called a patient presentation. What competent performance requires may now include more judgment.

Research on clinical expertise suggests that experience is associated with changes in how clinically relevant knowledge is organized and represented for use in patient problems (Norman, 2005; Schmidt & Rikers, 2007). These findings do not establish one universal sequence of learner development, but they help explain why competent clinical performance involves more than accumulating additional facts.

One place that difference may become visible is the patient presentation. A learner who was once mainly expected to gather and report may later be expected to select, interpret, and recommend.

Suppose you used to receive feedback that your presentations were thorough. Now your attending repeatedly interrupts and asks, "What do you think is going on?"

You could interpret that as evidence that a previously strong skill has deteriorated. Another possibility is that thoroughness is no longer sufficient for the current version of the task.

The question has changed from *Can you gather and report the information?* to *Can you decide which information matters and use it to make a judgment?*

That is a different problem to investigate. More practice reporting everything you know may not address it.

Independence: From Doing What You Are Told to Noticing What Needs Doing

Increasing responsibility can hide a similar shift. Early on, someone may tell you what to do next:

- *Check this result.*
- *Call this person.*
- *See this patient.*
- *Find out whether the medication was given.*

You can become very good at completing those tasks. Then the expectation may change.

Someone asks, "What needs to happen next?" Now the task includes recognizing the work before someone names it for you. You may need to notice that a result requires follow-up, decide which problem deserves attention first, or recognize that a change is important enough to bring to someone else.

The work has moved from completing prompted tasks toward identifying and prioritizing the tasks themselves. Increasing responsibility does not simply mean that supervision disappears. Entrustment scholarship treats responsibility as attached to particular professional activities and levels of supervision rather than as a global state of independence (ten Cate, 2013).

For this chapter, the practical point is narrower: **The activity may retain the same label while the amount of initiative or judgment expected within it changes.**

You may still be "following your patients." What that means at your current level may involve more anticipation, judgment, and initiative than it did several months ago.

That can produce an uncomfortable experience. You may be more capable than you were before and simultaneously less certain about whether you are doing enough.

The uncertainty does not establish that you are failing. It may tell you that you need to clarify what the current version of the task expects from you and where supervision remains appropriate.

Efficiency Works Until the Situation Requires Adaptation

There is another way the task can change. Sometimes you have developed a routine that works well, then encounter a situation where the routine no longer fits.

Familiar situations can reward efficiency. You recognize the pattern, know the sequence, and can perform without rebuilding the approach from the beginning each time.

A novel or changing situation may require something else. You need to notice that the familiar approach is insufficient and decide how to modify it.

Work on adaptive expertise has examined the tension between efficient use of familiar approaches and the need to adapt or learn when those approaches are insufficient for a new problem (Mylopoulos & Regehr, 2009; Mylopoulos & Woods, 2017). The student version can be much simpler. **A routine can be useful and still have an edge.**

You learn a reliable way to organize a straightforward patient presentation. Then you meet a patient with several interacting problems, and the same structure produces a confusing presentation.

The routine did not become worthless. The patient exposed a situation where the routine needed modification.

That is different from forgetting how to present. It is also different from claiming that every difficult case represents sophisticated adaptation.

The useful question is concrete: **What did this situation require that my usual approach did not provide?**

Look for the New Verb

A useful clue is to look for the new verb.

The task may still be called a presentation, but the work may have moved from reporting to selecting, interpreting, or recommending. You may still be studying, but the demand may have moved from recognizing to retrieving, discriminating, or applying. You may still be following your patients, but you are now expected not only to complete assigned tasks but to notice which tasks need attention.

The name can stay stable while the verbs underneath it change.

When that happens, comparing your current performance with an earlier version of the task can mislead you. You may not be performing the old task worse. You may be learning the newer one.

That possibility is not reassurance. It makes a prediction. If the demand has changed, practice aimed at the new verb should tell you more than simply repeating the old one.

A quick way to investigate the difficulty is to ask two questions:

- **What did competent performance require before?**
- **What does competent performance require now?**

Make the answer behavioral. "Be more advanced" tells you very little, while "state which diagnosis I favor and identify the findings that make it more likely than the alternatives" gives you something you can practice.

This also helps separate Chapter 3 from Chapter 2. **Chapter 2 asks where an expected performance broke down. Chapter 3 asks whether the expected performance itself changed.** Sometimes what looks like a failure of execution is the first sign that you have been practicing an earlier version of the task.

Test the Task-Change Hypothesis

The introduction gave you a distinction between a possible explanation and a working hypothesis. Use it here.

Suppose your current hypothesis is: *My presentations feel harder because I am now expected to prioritize and recommend, while I have mostly practiced gathering and reporting.*

Ask what you would expect to see if that explanation were useful. You might expect the history gathering itself to remain adequate while the assessment becomes the place where you hesitate.

You might also expect your presentations to become more focused when you practice stating the main problem, committing to an interpretation, and giving a recommendation before adding supporting detail. Then test it. On your next patient, try writing three lines before rounds:

- **What is the main problem?**
- **What do I think explains it?**
- **What do I think we should do next?**

Use those answers to organize the presentation. Then watch what happens.

If the presentation becomes more focused, that pattern supports the task-change hypothesis. If you cannot answer those three questions because you do not understand the patient's condition, Chapter 2 gives you a different explanation to investigate.

The same method works with studying. If you suspect the task now requires application rather than recognition alone, use practice that requires application and see where the performance fails.

With increasing responsibility, clarify what behaviors are actually expected at your current level. Then compare the clarified expectation with what you are already doing and where you still need support.

The purpose is not to prove that advancement explains every new difficulty. It is to find out whether you have been judging your current performance against an earlier version of the task.

Difficulty Is Not Evidence of Growth

There is an appealing story available here: if something feels harder, perhaps that means you are developing. Be careful with that conclusion. **Difficulty by itself does not prove which explanation is correct.**

A task may be difficult because you are encountering a more demanding version of the performance. It may also be difficult because you lack necessary knowledge, have not practiced enough, received unclear expectations, or are working under poor conditions.

Difficulty becomes informative when you examine what may be producing it, choose a response, and watch what happens next. Calling every difficulty developmental would make the explanation impossible to test.

The same standard from Chapter 2 applies. Ask what you would expect to change if your explanation were right.

If the task changed and you begin practicing the new demand, some part of your performance may eventually change too. If it does not, reopen the differential. You may need more knowledge, different practice, clearer feedback, or another explanation entirely.

Difficulty can create an opportunity to learn. It is not evidence that learning is occurring. Advancement is one possibility, not a universal reassurance.

Adaptability Is Not Accommodation to Dysfunction

There is another boundary worth keeping clear. Learning to adapt does not mean becoming increasingly skilled at tolerating every condition in which you are asked to work.

Some local practices are inefficient, confusing, poorly taught, or inadequately supported. Some environments create problems that should be addressed rather than absorbed by the learner.

The ability to modify your approach when a clinical problem changes is valuable. The ability to survive an unreasonable system without complaint is a different issue. **Adaptability is not accommodation to dysfunction.**

If the task has become harder because supervision, expectations, workload, or another condition is inappropriate, individual adaptation may not be the response the situation needs. Later chapters will examine those conditions more directly. Here, the boundary keeps the central argument honest: changing demands can require development, while the existence of a new demand does not automatically make that demand appropriate.

When the Name Stays the Same

You will encounter this pattern repeatedly in medical training. Familiar words may continue to describe work that asks something different of you than it did before.

Study may require more than recognizing what you have seen. *Present* may require more than reporting what you found. *Follow your patients* may come to include noticing what needs attention, forming judgments, and recognizing when someone else needs to become involved. The name stays stable while the verbs underneath it change.

That can make progress difficult to recognize. You may compare how effortless an earlier version became with how effortful the current version feels and conclude that you have moved backward.

Before reaching that conclusion, compare the tasks themselves. Ask what you were expected to do before and what you are expected to do now.

If the demands changed, identify the new behavior and practice that behavior directly. Then reassess whether the performance changes.

If the demands did not change, or if the difficulty persists after you have practiced the newer version of the task, reopen the differential. Another explanation may deserve more weight.

You did not necessarily become worse at something you had learned to do. **Sometimes you reached a version of the task that requires something new.**

Stabilizing Shift

If a task with a familiar name suddenly feels harder, look for the new verb hidden inside it.

You may not be doing the old task worse. You may be learning a version that asks more of you.

Options Menu

- **Compare the demands, not just the feeling.** Ask what competent performance required before, and what it requires now.
- **Test the task-change hypothesis.** Predict what should improve if the demand really changed, then practice that specific behavior and watch.
- **Write three lines before rounds.** State the main problem, what explains it, and what you would do next — then use those answers to organize the presentation.
- **Separate difficulty from growth.** Ask what would be different if this were actually a new demand, rather than assuming difficulty proves you are developing.

Common Trap

Treating difficulty as automatic proof of growth. This protects against feeling like something is wrong, but it can excuse a real gap in knowledge, practice, or feedback.

Treating adaptation as accommodation. Becoming skilled at tolerating a chaotic, undersupervised, or unsafe environment is not the same as developing. If the task became harder because of the conditions around it, the response may need to change the conditions, not just your tolerance for them.

Recap

What to remember when stressed:

- A task can demand something new without changing its name — look for the new verb.
- Comparing yourself to an earlier version of the task can mislead you if the task itself changed.
- Test the task-change hypothesis: predict what should improve, then practice and watch.
- Difficulty is not evidence of growth, and adaptability is not accommodation to dysfunction.
- If the demands did not change, or the difficulty persists, reopen the differential.

PART II

What Does the Evidence Actually Tell You?

Medical school gives you a remarkable amount of information about your performance. The harder problem is deciding how much that information actually tells you.

You finish a presentation feeling terrible, and your resident says nothing about it. An attending corrects your assessment twice, another student seems much faster, or an evaluation contains one sentence you read six times trying to determine how worried you should be.

Sometimes the information is reassuring. A supervisor tells you that you are progressing appropriately, your scores improve, or a task that once required constant help becomes increasingly reliable.

Even then, your internal experience may tell a different story. You can have evidence that you are progressing while still feeling uncertain, or feel increasingly comfortable while an important weakness remains unresolved.

Part II is about learning to work with that disagreement. The central question is no longer simply *How do I think I am doing?*

It is: **What does the evidence I have reasonably allow me to conclude?**

Chapter 4 begins with your own experience. It asks how much weight to give a difficult day, a feeling of confidence or uncertainty, a repeated pattern, and your trajectory over time.

Chapter 5 turns to another person's observation. Feedback becomes more useful when you can identify what someone actually observed, what they concluded from it, and what that information supports doing next.

Chapter 6 asks about the expectations and standards underneath the judgment. A comment such as "be more concise" means little until you understand what competent concision looks like in that setting and whether the expectation being applied is appropriate for your level.

These are three different evidence problems. Your experience tells you something about what the performance felt like. Feedback tells you something about what another person observed and interpreted. Expectations help determine what the performance was being judged against.

Together, they give you a more disciplined way to interpret what a difficult performance means. One principle will run through all three chapters: **The larger the conclusion, the more evidence it should require.**

A single difficult presentation may tell you something important about that presentation. By itself, it usually cannot establish that you are behind, unready, bad at clinical medicine, or in the wrong profession.

That principle works in both directions. Feeling confident does not establish readiness, and feeling unready does not establish that you are unprepared. Confidence and competence are related but distinct, and their alignment can vary with the task, the learner, and the surrounding context (Gottlieb et al., 2022).

The goal is proportionality. **The size of the conclusion should stay close to the strength, consistency, and relevance of the evidence supporting it.**

Part II will therefore ask you to stop demanding competence verdicts from information that cannot provide them. You do not need to ignore weak or incomplete evidence. You do need to stop asking it to support conclusions larger than it can carry.

CHAPTER FOUR

Am I Actually Doing Okay?

You finish presenting a new patient, and your resident says, "Okay." She turns back to the computer, enters an order, and starts talking with the pharmacist.

Ten minutes later, the other medical student presents. When he finishes, the same resident says, "Nice job," before the team moves on. You know two words are not an evaluation. By lunch, you may still be wondering what they mean.

Then you start supplying your own evidence. You hesitated before giving the differential, forgot one laboratory result, and needed a prompt before committing to the plan. You also saw the patient independently, and your resident did not correct most of what you said. Depending on where your mind is already leaning, either fact can begin to feel diagnostic.

This is where self-assessment becomes difficult. You have direct access to your own uncertainty, effort, hesitation, mistakes, and relief, but experiencing the performance directly does not tell you automatically what caused it or what it means. Do not ignore how you feel, but **do not ask the feeling to identify its own cause.**

Your Experience Is Evidence

Suppose you walk away from rounds thinking, *I felt completely lost.* That feeling matters because it tells you something about your experience of the task.

Perhaps you were working at the edge of what you could manage independently. Maybe you could not organize the information quickly enough, or perhaps you were unsure what your supervisor expected from you. The feeling can direct your attention toward something worth investigating. What it cannot do by itself is tell you which explanation is correct.

This distinction is important because dismissing subjective experience would create its own problem. You are often the only person who knows how effortful a performance felt, where you hesitated, which decisions felt uncertain, and how much help you needed to reach the answer.

Those observations can be useful. The mistake occurs when the experience becomes its own explanation. *I felt lost* can become *I performed badly*, which can become *I am behind*, which can become *I am not ready for this.* Each step enlarges the conclusion without necessarily adding evidence.

Work on self-assessment in the health professions has repeatedly questioned the accuracy and usefulness of broad, decontextualized judgments of one's own competence. More recent review work continues to identify substantial limitations in using global self-assessment as a proxy for competence, while Eva and Regehr distinguish those broad judgments from more situation-specific self-monitoring—awareness of whether one has the knowledge or skill needed for a particular problem (Eva & Regehr, 2005, 2011; Yates et al., 2022).

The practical lesson is narrower: **Your experience belongs in the evidence. It should not be asked to settle the case alone.** For this book, it helps to sort performance evidence at three levels: event, pattern, and trajectory.

Event

Start with what actually happened. *I felt terrible during that presentation* describes your experience of an event. *My presentation was terrible* has already moved from experience toward judgment.

Get more specific. Perhaps you spent four minutes recounting the history before reaching the assessment, or your attending asked for your differential twice before you gave one.

Maybe you proposed a plan but could not explain why you preferred it. Perhaps you answered most of the questions accurately and became preoccupied with the one answer you missed. These descriptions do not eliminate interpretation. They make the event specific enough to examine.

That matters because a specific event can support a specific response. *I am bad at presentations* gives you almost nothing to work on, while *I repeatedly delayed stating my assessment until someone prompted me* identifies something observable.

The event may matter a great deal. A single safety-critical mistake, for example, can require immediate attention without waiting for a pattern to emerge. For many ordinary developmental questions, however, one event supports a smaller conclusion. It tells you what happened once under a particular set of conditions.

Pattern

Now ask whether the same thing keeps happening. Suppose three different supervisors have told you that your presentations contain the relevant information but make it difficult to identify the main clinical problem.

That is different evidence from one attending interrupting one presentation. The pattern becomes more informative when the observations are reasonably specific and concern similar performances.

"Needs improvement" repeated three times still leaves important questions unanswered, while three observations that you delay committing to an assessment point toward something more interpretable. Patterns can also appear in your own observations.

You may notice that you understand material when studying but repeatedly struggle to retrieve it without cues, or that you consistently lose track of your plan when a presentation is interrupted. Chapter 2 gives you the differential for investigating those problems. Chapter 4 asks a different question: **How much evidence do I have that this is actually a recurring problem?**

A repeated, reasonably consistent pattern usually gives you more to work with than one memorable event. It still needs interpretation, and the quality of the observations matters.

Trajectory

A pattern tells you what has been happening. Trajectory asks what direction the pattern is moving. Imagine that your first several presentations require frequent prompting. Over the next two weeks, you begin reaching the assessment sooner, need fewer prompts, and receive more specific responsibility for presenting the plan.

You may still feel uncomfortable. The task may still require substantial effort, and you may continue noticing every hesitation. The trajectory nevertheless contains information that the feeling alone does not: something about the performance is changing.

Now imagine the opposite. You have received the same specific feedback several times, practiced the skill in a way intended to address it, and continue making the same error without meaningful improvement. That trajectory matters too. It gives you reason to revisit the explanation, the intervention, or both.

For developmental questions, comparing performances over time can reveal information that one snapshot cannot. Trajectory does not make every upward line reassuring or every plateau concerning. It gives you another piece of evidence with which to judge whether a problem is changing, persisting, or becoming clearer.

Conclusion

Only after looking at the event, pattern, and trajectory should you ask how large a conclusion the evidence can reasonably support. This is where the proportionality rule becomes important: **The larger the conclusion, the more evidence it should require.**

I missed an important finding in this patient is a conclusion about an event. *I repeatedly miss important findings in similar patients* describes a pattern. *I am behind* is much larger. So are *I am not ready*, *I am bad at this*, and *I do not belong here.*

Those conclusions reach beyond one performance into judgments about your broader competence, developmental position, or identity. They therefore require more evidence than one painful event can usually provide. **Do not make the conclusion larger than the evidence supporting it.**

Confidence and Readiness Can Disagree

Consider two students preparing for a high-stakes examination. Student A feels unready. Practice questions remain effortful, and every missed item seems to expose another thing she does not know.

Her performance evidence tells a fuller story. Across repeated assessments, her performance has improved, she is meeting the relevant benchmarks being used to judge readiness, and the specific weaknesses identified earlier are becoming less frequent.

Her feeling of unreadiness still matters. It may identify areas she wants to review or tell her that the stakes feel high. It does not erase the trajectory. **Feeling unready and having evidence of inadequate readiness are different findings.**

Student B feels increasingly comfortable. The material looks familiar, studying moves quickly, and many explanations feel obvious when he reads them. His performance data tell a different story.

Across repeated assessments, the same type of reasoning error persists, and targeted practice has not yet changed it. His growing familiarity is real. It is also insufficient evidence that the unresolved weakness has disappeared.

Neither student needs to treat confidence as a verdict. Both can ask what the feeling adds to the other evidence available. This is why confidence and readiness are not interchangeable.

Confidence is part of the evidence about your experience. Readiness requires evidence about what you can actually do under the relevant conditions.

Evidence Before Verdict

When you notice yourself reaching a large conclusion after a difficult performance, it may help to spend five minutes separating the conclusion from the evidence underneath it. Try pairing what you feel or fear with what evidence you actually have.

- **"I am behind."** The evidence: my attending corrected my assessment twice today.
- **"I am terrible at presentations."** The evidence: I needed prompting to state the main problem on two patients.
- **"Everyone else is more ready than I am."** The evidence: another student answered three questions I could not answer.

Do not use the second column to argue with the first. Use it to determine what you actually know.

Then ask three questions: **Is this an event, a pattern, or a trajectory? How large a conclusion can this evidence support? What additional evidence would meaningfully change my conclusion?**

That final question matters. Sometimes you do not need more analysis of the evidence you already have. **You need another observation.**

You may need to ask a supervisor whether the problem they noticed is isolated or recurring, compare several performances, or see what happens after targeted practice. The goal is **Evidence Before Verdict**, a short practice for moments when the conclusion has become larger than the information underneath it.

Ask for Information That Can Answer the Question

Sometimes the evidence gap is external. Nobody has told you that you are struggling, but nobody has given you enough specific information to know how your performance compares with expectations either.

Silence does not solve that problem. **Silence is missing information, not proof of failure or proof that everything is fine.**

You can ask for something more interpretable: "What's one thing I'm doing at the expected level and one thing I should change on my next shift?" The question is bounded enough to answer and specific enough to give you information about current performance. Chapter 5 will examine what to do with the answer once you receive it.

For now, notice the purpose of asking. You are not requesting reassurance. You are obtaining evidence that can help answer a question your mood, your resident's facial expression, or one difficult presentation cannot settle.

Let Evidence Update You in Both Directions

Calibration requires allowing your conclusion to change when the evidence changes. Sometimes that means taking a concern more seriously. A repeated, specific weakness observed across performances deserves more attention than *I was just having a bad day* can provide.

Sometimes the update goes the other way. If people who have repeatedly observed your work tell you that you are performing appropriately for your level and your trajectory supports that judgment, continuing to reject that evidence because the work still feels difficult does not make the judgment more accurate.

The goal is not reassurance. **The goal is proportionality between the evidence and the conclusion.**

Your feelings remain part of that evidence. They may tell you that a task is effortful, unfamiliar, frightening, or important to you.

Instead, move outward. What happened in this event, and has it happened repeatedly? What direction is the performance moving? What direct observations do you have, and what important information is still missing?

Then decide how large a conclusion the evidence can carry. **Big conclusions still have to earn their size.**

You may discover something that needs work. You may discover that the evidence supports more readiness than you feel. Either result is useful because Chapter 4 is not trying to make you feel better about your performance. It is trying to help you draw conclusions that are **proportional to the evidence.**

Stabilizing Shift

Before deciding what a difficult moment means, separate the finding from the feeling: what actually happened, and what conclusion you are tempted to draw from it.

Use this as a flashlight, not a courtroom. You are looking for the next useful piece of information, not building a case against yourself.

Options Menu

- **Sort by Event, Pattern, or Trajectory.** One bad moment is an event. Three similar corrections are a pattern. Change over time is a trajectory — each deserves a different-sized conclusion.
- **Pair feeling with evidence.** Write down what you feel or fear next to what evidence you actually have, and use the second column to test the first, not confirm it.
- **Ask a bounded question.** Try "What's one thing I'm doing well and one thing I should change?" — specific enough to answer, useful enough to act on.
- **Let the evidence update you both ways.** If people who have watched you consistently say you are ready, that convergence is evidence too, not just reassurance.

Common Trap

Treating a single difficult moment as proof of a stable trait — "I am terrible at this" — when the same evidence would only support a narrower, more specific conclusion. This protects you from feeling caught off guard, but it makes the conclusion far larger than the evidence can carry.

A calmer alternative: match the size of your conclusion to the size of the evidence — an event supports a narrower claim than a trajectory does.

Recap

What to remember when stressed:

- Separate the event, the pattern, and the trajectory before deciding what a difficult moment means.
- Your own experience is evidence, but not the only evidence — pair it with what you can observe.
- Confidence and readiness can disagree; ask which one the evidence actually supports.
- If the evidence is missing, ask a bounded question rather than guessing.
- The larger the conclusion, the more evidence it should require.

CHAPTER FIVE

What Does the Feedback Actually Tell You?

Your attending listens to your presentation, asks two questions about the plan, and says, "You need to take more ownership." You nod. The phrase sounds important, and you write it down later because you do not want to dismiss feedback simply because you do not immediately understand it. Then you try to figure out what to do differently tomorrow.

Should you see your patients earlier, make more decisions without asking your resident, volunteer for more tasks, speak with greater confidence, or know more about every problem on the list? The feedback has given you a conclusion without enough information about the observation behind it. *Take more ownership* may point toward something important, but until you know what behavior produced the judgment, you cannot tell what needs to change.

That is the problem this chapter addresses. Feedback is evidence, but what it can tell you depends partly on the observation underneath it and the context in which that observation was made.

Chapter 4 asked how large a conclusion your evidence could support. Chapter 5 asks what happens when some of that evidence comes from another person—and how much that evidence can reasonably carry.

Feedback Is an Interpretation of a Performance

Feedback can feel more authoritative than your own impression because it comes from outside you. Someone else watched you work and reached a conclusion.

That external perspective matters. Supervisors can notice things you cannot see while you are performing, and they may know expectations you are still learning.

Their perspective is still a perspective. What they communicate includes both an observation and an interpretation of what that observation means.

Consider the difference between these statements:

- "You need to be more confident."
- "When I asked which diagnosis you thought was most likely, you gave three possibilities but did not tell me which one you favored."

The first describes a quality the observer thinks you should have more of. The second describes something you did.

That distinction matters because several behaviors could produce the impression of low confidence. You might speak quietly, hedge every recommendation, avoid committing to an assessment, look down while answering, or ask for confirmation after decisions you are already expected to make.

Those are different behaviors. They may have different causes and require different responses, so a useful first move with feedback is to ask: **What did this person actually observe?**

Translate Traits Back Into Behavior

Medical feedback often arrives in language that sounds like a description of the learner rather than the performance:

- *Be more confident.*
- *Take more ownership.*
- *Be more efficient.*
- *Work on your clinical reasoning.*

Each phrase may contain useful information. None tells you precisely what to do next.

Suppose your resident says, "You need to take more ownership." Compare that with: "Before rounds tomorrow, review the overnight results and tell me which changes affect today's plan."

The second statement translates the broad judgment into observable behavior. You now know what the supervisor expected and what performance you can attempt tomorrow.

The same translation works with other feedback. *Be more confident* might become: "When you have enough information to form an assessment, state which diagnosis you favor before listing the alternatives."

Be more efficient might become: "On stable follow-up patients, lead with the active problem instead of repeating the full history." *Work on your clinical reasoning* might become: "When you give your differential, tell me which finding makes your first diagnosis more likely than your second."

The translation does not prove that the supervisor's interpretation was correct. It makes the interpretation specific enough to examine. The central move is to translate trait-like feedback into observable behavior, then examine what the feedback actually supports.

Observation → Meaning → Next Move

Three questions can keep feedback from becoming a global verdict:

- **What did they observe?**
- **What did they think it meant?**
- **What could I change or test next?**

Start with the observation. If your attending says you need to be more efficient, ask what part of the performance created that impression.

Perhaps your presentations consistently take longer than expected because you include information that does not affect the current plan. Now you have an observable performance to work with.

Then consider meaning. The extra detail might reflect difficulty prioritizing, uncertainty about the expected presentation style, or a habit that has persisted from an earlier stage of training.

Chapter 2 gives you a way to distinguish among those explanations. The feedback identifies a performance that deserves investigation; it does not necessarily identify the cause.

Finally, identify the next move. You might practice giving the assessment first, ask your resident which information they would leave out, or set a specific target for tomorrow's presentations.

Feedback becomes more useful when it gives you something observable to change or test on the next attempt—and when there is another opportunity to use what you learned. Workplace-feedback research increasingly treats feedback as a process that extends beyond receiving information to acting on it in subsequent work (Fuentes-Cimma et al., 2024). A label tells you what someone thought; a behavioral translation gives you something to investigate.

Ask for the Observation Underneath the Label

You will not always receive feedback in its most useful form. Sometimes you may need to help make it more specific.

If someone says "be more confident," you can ask: "What did you notice me doing that gave you that impression?"

If the feedback is "take more ownership," you might ask: "What's one thing you expected me to do today that I didn't do?"

If you hear "work on your clinical reasoning," try: "Can you point to one place in my assessment where you wanted me to reason differently?"

These questions do not challenge the supervisor to defend the evaluation. They ask for the information you need to use it.

Sometimes the answer will clarify the issue immediately. "You knew the plan, but you waited for me to say it before you recommended it" gives you far more to work with than "be more confident."

Sometimes the supervisor will struggle to provide an example. That tells you something about the specificity of the evidence available, although it does not automatically make the original impression wrong.

Your task is to determine what the feedback can reasonably support. Chapter 4's proportionality rule still applies: **the larger the conclusion, the more evidence it should require.**

Not Every Observer Sees the Same Performance

One attending tells you that your presentations need more detail. The next tells you to stop giving so much detail.

This can feel contradictory until you ask what each person actually observed and what standard each was applying. One may have watched you present a new admission, while the other heard you present a stable follow-up patient.

The feedback may also reflect different legitimate preferences. Supervisors can value different forms of organization, communication, initiative, and efficiency even when they are observing the same learner.

Research in medical education suggests that learners do not simply receive feedback as neutral information. They make judgments about its credibility, and systematic review evidence indicates that those judgments can be shaped by the characteristics of the feedback, its context, the perceived credibility of the source, and characteristics of the recipient (Watling et al., 2012; Telio et al., 2015, 2016; Dai et al., 2021).

Feedback is neither objective truth nor merely personal opinion. It is information generated by an observer encountering a performance in a particular context, and both the observation and the meaning assigned to it can vary with the assessor, the task, and the situation (Gingerich et al., 2014).

How Much Weight Should This Feedback Carry?

Suppose a supervisor who watched one presentation tells you that your clinical reasoning is weak. The comment matters, but the breadth of the conclusion exceeds what one presentation can easily establish.

Now suppose several supervisors who have directly observed you across several patients independently identify the same specific problem. Each notes that you generate reasonable differentials but struggle to identify which findings distinguish your leading diagnoses.

That pattern gives you more to work with than the isolated comment. The observations are specific, repeated across performances, and similar enough to ask whether they are identifying the same problem.

When deciding how much weight to give feedback, ask whether the person was in a position to observe the performance they are commenting on. Ask whether they had enough opportunity to see the relevant behavior and whether the information is specific enough that you can identify what they were reacting to.

Then look for similar observations across performances or observers. The observer's understanding of the task, context, and expected level may also affect how useful their interpretation is.

None of these questions makes an observer infallible. They help you decide how much work a particular piece of feedback can reasonably do.

When Feedback Conflicts

Conflicting feedback does not always mean one person is right and the other is wrong. Sometimes the observers saw different performances or were responding to different parts of the task.

Return to the observations first. Suppose one attending says your presentations are too detailed and another says they need more detail.

Ask which patients they heard you present, which parts they wanted changed, and what information each considered necessary for the task. You may discover that the apparent conflict becomes smaller once the observations are specific.

One supervisor may have wanted a shorter history, while the other wanted a clearer explanation of the assessment. Those comments are compatible: you can reduce irrelevant detail and increase clinically important reasoning at the same time.

Sometimes the conflict is real. Two supervisors may genuinely prefer different approaches, or they may apply different expectations to the same performance.

In those cases, the next question is not simply which supervisor is correct. Ask what appears portable, what may be local, and what each person counted as good performance.

That last question leads directly into Chapter 6. Conflicting feedback often becomes more interpretable once you can see the standard underneath each judgment.

Take the Feedback Into the Next Attempt

Feedback becomes more useful when it gives you something to test on the next attempt. Suppose you receive the comment: *"Your assessment needs to be stronger."* Translated, the observation might be that you listed four diagnoses without saying which one you favored; the next move is to state your leading diagnosis and its strongest support before discussing alternatives.

That translation makes a prediction. If the problem was that your reasoning stayed hidden, making it explicit should change what the supervisor sees next — the assessment should become easier to follow, and the same feedback should stop repeating. If it does not, revisit what the feedback meant or whether another part of the performance is breaking down.

The process is iterative. **Feedback helps you choose a next attempt, and the next attempt generates more evidence.**

When the Feedback Is Poor

Some feedback will remain vague despite your efforts to clarify it. Some will arrive too late, reflect limited observation, or provide a judgment without enough information to make the judgment useful.

Occasionally, feedback may be delivered in a humiliating, discriminatory, retaliatory, or otherwise harmful way. The educational value of a comment does not make harmful conduct acceptable.

An elaborate framework is not necessary for every instance. What matters is separating whatever usable information exists from the way it was delivered, while also seeking appropriate support when the interaction or pattern requires it.

A poorly delivered comment can still contain a useful observation. A harmful interaction can also require attention beyond extracting a lesson from it.

The important distinction is between the authority of the person giving feedback and the quality of the evidence contained in the feedback. One does not automatically establish the other.

When the Evidence Converges

There is an opposite problem worth naming. You can contextualize each comment so thoroughly that repeated concerning information never changes the working hypothesis.

One attending prefers a different style. Another only saw you on a difficult day. A third has not worked with you for long.

Any of those explanations may be true. They do not make a repeated, specific pattern irrelevant if one begins to emerge.

Suppose several supervisors have directly observed you and independently identify the same specific difficulty. You clarify what they mean, work on the behavior, and the problem continues to appear.

That convergence deserves attention. When repeated, specific observations continue to point toward the same difficulty, let that pattern change the working hypothesis rather than explaining each observation away separately.

Return to the Developmental Differential and ask what explains the persistent performance and what kind of response the evidence now supports. You may need more knowledge, coached practice, clearer expectations, closer supervision, or further assessment.

The point is to use the evidence rather than protect a preferred conclusion from it. Context matters, but context should not make the explanation impossible to revise.

What Standard Was Being Applied?

Feedback contains a comparison even when the comparison remains invisible. *Too slow* compared with what, and *not enough ownership* for which level of training?

Too detailed may mean too detailed for this attending, this clinical situation, or competent performance more generally. *Needs stronger reasoning* raises the same question: according to which expected behavior?

Those questions matter because you cannot fully interpret an observation until you understand what the observer expected instead. Chapter 5 has asked you to recover the observation, decide what that observation can reasonably support, and identify what to test next. Chapter 6 adds the question underneath the judgment: **What standard was being applied?**

Stabilizing Shift

Before deciding what feedback means, ask what your supervisor actually observed — a trait-like label such as "be more confident" describes an impression, not a behavior you can practice.

Options Menu

- **Translate the trait into behavior.** Ask what specific action the label is standing in for, then practice that behavior directly.
- **Ask for the observation underneath the label.** Try "What did you notice me doing that gave you that impression?"
- **Weigh the feedback before acting on it.** One comment from someone who watched you once carries less weight than a pattern several supervisors independently describe.
- **Take it into your next attempt.** Turn the feedback into a prediction — if the translation is right, a specific next performance should look different.

Common Trap

Treating a single piece of feedback as either the whole truth or worth dismissing entirely, depending on how much it stings.

How much feedback hurts and how much evidence it carries are two different questions.

A calmer alternative: ask what was actually observed, then decide how much weight the observation deserves.

Recap

What to remember when stressed:

- Feedback is an interpretation of a performance, not the performance itself.
- Translate trait-like language ("be more confident") into observable behavior before acting on it.
- Ask what was observed, what it was thought to mean, and what you could change or test next.
- Weight feedback by how directly it was observed and whether it converges across supervisors.
- When feedback conflicts, look at what each person actually saw before deciding who is right.

CHAPTER SIX

The Rules Nobody Told You

You finish presenting a patient, and your attending says, "You don't need to tell me all of that." Yesterday, another attending stopped you because you had left out details she wanted to hear. You adjusted after that conversation, so today you included them. Now the same behavior is being corrected in the opposite direction.

You know how to present a patient. What you do not yet know is what counts as a good presentation to this person, on this service, for this kind of patient.

That distinction matters because evaluative feedback implies some standard of comparison, even when the standard is not stated. When someone tells you that you were too detailed, too passive, too slow, insufficiently prepared, or not independent enough, the judgment depends on an expectation about what competent performance should have looked like instead.

Sometimes that expectation is clear and appropriate for your level. Sometimes it is legitimate but has never been explained, and sometimes it reflects a local preference that will change with the next supervisor. Occasionally, the expectation itself is inappropriate. Before you can use the feedback well, you need to know **what standard was actually being applied.**

You Know the Medicine. You Do Not Yet Know How Medicine Is Done Here.

Imagine starting a new inpatient service. You know how to review a chart, take a history, examine a patient, and organize a presentation.

By the end of the first morning, you have also learned that knowing how to do those things does not tell you exactly how this team expects them to be done. Your resident expects you to check the overnight nursing notes before rounds. Your attending wants the assessment immediately after the one-liner, while another attending on the same service prefers to hear the new data first. The fellow expects students to call consultants only after discussing the question with the team. Nobody told you any of this when the rotation started.

Chapter 1 asked what happens when a new environment changes the work around you. The question here is narrower: **What counted as good performance in this environment?**

Clinical learning involves more than applying knowledge in a new location. Medical students also learn through participation in clinical practice, including through observation and progressively more active involvement in the work (Dornan et al., 2007).

The practical problem is not simply that an expectation was unstated. It is determining what kind of expectation you encountered and how much of it should travel with you.

Not Every Unwritten Rule Is the Same

Suppose your attending tells you that you should have called about a new result instead of waiting until rounds. Before deciding what the correction means about your performance, ask what kind of expectation was involved.

Some expectations are **explicit standards** appropriate to your level. You were told that certain changes should be communicated immediately, and the expectation was reasonable for the responsibility you had been given.

Others are **tacit workplace expectations**. Everyone on the service may know that a particular result needs to be reviewed before rounds, but nobody realized that a new student would not know the routine.

Some are **local preferences**. One attending wants presentations organized by problem, while another prefers a more traditional sequence.

Others reflect a **broader cultural or institutional norm**. A hospital, specialty, or training program may have established ways of communicating, escalating concerns, documenting decisions, or dividing responsibilities.

Finally, some expectations are **inappropriate**. Being expected to tolerate humiliation, conceal uncertainty that affects patient safety, work outside appropriate supervision, or accept discriminatory treatment does not become legitimate because the expectation is common or unspoken.

These categories can overlap, and you will not always know immediately which one you are dealing with. The distinction still matters because **invisible does not mean illegitimate, and familiar does not mean appropriate.**

Explicit Standards

The easiest case is a standard that has been clearly communicated. Your resident tells you on the first day, "If one of your patients develops a new oxygen requirement, let me know when you find out rather than waiting until rounds."

The next morning, you notice a new oxygen requirement and decide to wait because rounds begin in twenty minutes. Your resident later tells you that you should have called.

There is relatively little mystery about the standard. You knew what was expected and did not meet it.

The useful question is therefore not *Why didn't anyone tell me the rules?* You were told. Now you need to understand why the expected behavior did not occur.

Perhaps you underestimated the significance of the change, forgot the instruction, or were uncertain whether this situation met the threshold your resident had described. That returns you to Chapter 2. **An unclear standard and a clearly communicated standard you have not met are different problems.**

This distinction keeps Chapter 6 from becoming a way to explain every correction as a communication failure. Sometimes the expectation was visible, appropriate, and still missed.

Legitimate Expectations That Nobody Made Explicit

Now change the situation. Nobody told you that the team expects students to notify the resident about certain new results before rounds.

You discover the expectation when your resident asks, "Why didn't you tell me about this earlier?" The correction still contains useful information: the team has identified a behavior it expects in this situation.

The difference is that you were being evaluated against a standard you had not yet been given a reasonable opportunity to know. You still need to learn the expectation, but the fact that the standard was tacit matters when you interpret the original performance.

You may therefore be learning the task while simultaneously discovering some of the criteria by which the task is being judged. Once a legitimate expectation becomes visible, you can use it. Ask what situations trigger the behavior, what level of independence is expected, and whether the rule applies broadly or only in particular circumstances.

You do not need every detail of a workplace explained before you participate. The useful distinction is whether a performance judgment depended partly on information you were still acquiring about how the workplace functions.

Local Preferences Are Still Information

Some rules are narrower. One attending wants every relevant laboratory result included in the presentation. Another stops you after the sodium and says, "I can read the labs. Tell me what matters."

Neither preference necessarily establishes the universal form of a good presentation. Both tell you something about how a particular supervisor wants information communicated.

That information can still be useful. Adapting communication to the person and situation is part of functioning in clinical work.

The problem begins when a local preference becomes a global verdict. *Dr. Patel wants shorter presentations* is different from *I am bad at presenting patients.*

When you are unsure which kind of standard you have encountered, ask: **Would another reasonable supervisor consider this part of competent performance at my level, or is this primarily a local preference?**

You may not always know the answer. Asking the question prevents one person's style from automatically becoming your definition of competence.

You can also ask directly: "Is that something you'd recommend I do generally, or is it how you prefer presentations on this service?" A thoughtful supervisor may tell you that the expectation is broadly important, specific to the clinical situation, or simply a preference. Any of those answers gives you better evidence than guessing.

Institutional and Cultural Norms

Some expectations extend beyond one supervisor. You may enter a service where students routinely call consultants, while another service expects those conversations to go through residents. One institution may expect particular concerns to be escalated through a defined chain, while another organizes responsibility differently.

These norms can matter even when nobody thinks to explain them. People who have worked in the environment for years may no longer recognize which parts of their routine are obvious only because they have become familiar.

That is part of what makes tacit expectations difficult for newcomers. The learner sees unexplained behaviors while established members may experience them as simply how the work gets done.

Hidden-curriculum scholarship draws attention to lessons and messages conveyed outside the formal curriculum, including through the structures, relationships, practices, and culture of medical education (Hafferty & Franks, 1994; Lawrence et al., 2018). That does not make every unexplained local preference part of the hidden curriculum. For the learner, the practical question remains concrete: **Is this expectation telling me something about competent practice, something about how this institution organizes the work, or something about one person's preferred way of doing it?**

Those answers can overlap. You still want to know which part of the lesson should travel with you when you leave.

Make the Tacit Explicit

You cannot ask about every possible rule before a rotation begins. You can clarify the expectations most likely to affect your work.

Early in a new setting, a few questions can reveal a great deal:

- "What does a strong presentation look like to you?"
- "What should I make sure I know before rounds?"
- "Which decisions should I make myself, and which should I run by you?"
- "Are there changes you want me to tell you about immediately?"
- "How do you prefer students to ask for feedback?"

These questions are useful because they ask for behavior rather than personality. "What does a good student do?" invites a broad judgment, while "Which decisions should I run by you?" clarifies a usable expectation.

Choose the questions whose answers will change what you do; the rest can wait. Observation helps too. Watch what supervisors consistently correct, what experienced team members communicate without prompting, and which behaviors appear to matter across several people rather than only one. Then check your interpretation when the distinction matters. The goal is to make the consequential parts of the standard visible enough to use without trying to decode every preference of every clinical team.

When Feedback Conflicts, Look Underneath It

Chapter 5 asked what someone actually observed. Chapter 6 adds another question: **What did they expect instead?**

Suppose one supervisor tells you to show more initiative, while another tells you that you are acting too independently. Those comments appear contradictory until you know what behaviors each person saw and what responsibility each expected you to carry.

Perhaps the first wanted you to propose a plan before asking what to do. The second wanted you to discuss the plan before placing an order.

Now the apparent contradiction contains a more useful distinction. You are expected to form a judgment independently while still checking certain actions before carrying them out.

The standard becomes clearer when you separate **thinking, proposing, and acting**. What initially sounded like incompatible feedback may describe different points along the same task.

Sometimes the conflict will remain because supervisors can have genuinely different preferences. In those cases, distinguish what appears portable from what appears local, then adapt the local behavior when doing so is reasonable.

When the Standard Itself Is the Problem

Learning local expectations is part of entering a workplace. That does not require accepting every expectation as legitimate.

Suppose a learner discovers that asking questions is routinely mocked, uncertainty is treated as weakness, or students are pressured to take responsibility beyond the supervision appropriate to their role. The fact that these expectations are socially enforced does not make them educationally or professionally sound. The same is true of discriminatory expectations, humiliation, retaliation, or practices that compromise safety.

A learner may need to understand that these conditions exist without accepting responsibility for repairing or accommodating them alone. This is where the question *What standard was being applied?* becomes more than a way to improve performance. It allows you to examine the standard itself.

Ask whether the expectation is appropriate for your level and responsibility, whether it supports safe participation and learning, and whether it is consistent with broader expectations rather than simply normalized in one environment. When the answer is unclear and the stakes matter, you might seek perspective from an appropriate supervisor, advisor, program resource, or other trusted channel. Students can seek clarity without becoming responsible for repairing poorly designed or harmful learning environments.

Normalization does not make an expectation appropriate. A learner can correctly identify a local rule and still conclude that the rule should not be accepted as a legitimate standard.

What Should Travel With You?

By the end of a rotation, you will have learned many ways of doing things. Some may become part of how you work, while others may stay behind when you leave.

A supervisor may teach you a clearer way to present an assessment that improves your communication across settings. That lesson may be portable.

You may also learn that one attending wants laboratory values reported in a particular order. You can adapt while working with that attending without treating the preference as a universal standard.

Another experience may teach you something about the institution rather than the individual. You may learn how responsibility is divided, where to find help, or which communication route is used when something needs urgent attention.

The task is not simply to absorb every rule. It is to tell an explicit standard from a tacit expectation, a local preference, an institutional norm, and an inappropriate demand — then ask how portable the lesson is.

That distinction protects you from two opposite mistakes. You do not want to dismiss every correction as *just their preference*, and you do not want every supervisor's preference to become evidence that you were previously doing medicine wrong.

What standard was being applied? tells you what you encountered.

How much of it should travel with me? tells you what to do with it.

What Counted as Good Performance Here?

Part II began with your experience. Chapter 4 asked how large a conclusion that experience could reasonably support. Chapter 5 added another person's observation and asked what the feedback actually told you.

Now Chapter 6 has made the comparison underneath that feedback visible. A judgment requires a standard.

Before you use that judgment to reach a conclusion about your competence, ask what standard was being applied and what kind of standard it was. Sometimes the answer will be straightforward. The expectation was clear, appropriate, and you did not meet it. Take that information seriously and investigate what prevented the expected performance. **An**

unclear standard and a clearly communicated standard you have not met are different problems.

Sometimes you were still discovering a legitimate feature of the workplace. Learn it, clarify what matters, and watch whether the performance changes once the expectation becomes visible.

Sometimes you are encountering a local preference. Adapt where appropriate without turning the preference into a universal verdict about your ability.

Sometimes the standard itself deserves scrutiny. A rule does not become legitimate merely because nobody wrote it down or because everyone around you has learned to live with it.

The question that began Part II was *What does the evidence actually tell you?* By now, you have three ways to approach it: ask what your experience supports, ask what another person actually observed, and ask what standard they were using to interpret what they saw.

Together, those questions make performance evidence more legible. Before deciding what a judgment says about you, find out **what counted as good performance in the first place—and how much of that standard should travel with you.**

Stabilizing Shift

Before deciding what a correction means about you, ask what kind of standard you just encountered — an explicit rule, a local preference, or something that was never actually taught.

Options Menu

- **Ask a few questions early.** Try "What does a strong presentation look like to you?" or "Which decisions should I make myself, and which should I run by you?"
- **Test whether it is a preference or a standard.** Ask yourself: would another reasonable supervisor consider this part of competent performance at my level?
- **Separate thinking, proposing, and executing.** When feedback conflicts, the disagreement is often about which piece of the task each supervisor expects you to own.
- **Decide what should travel with you.** Some lessons are genuinely transferable skills; others are one attending's preference or one institution's local culture.

Common Trap

Assuming every uncorrected mistake means you should have already known the rule — when some expectations are tacit, local, or simply never communicated. This protects a sense that the system is fair and legible, but it can turn an ordinary gap in orientation into a verdict about your competence.

A calmer alternative: ask whether the standard was ever actually made available to you before deciding what failing to meet it means.

Recap

What to remember when stressed:

- Not every unwritten rule is the same kind of thing: explicit standard, tacit expectation, local preference, institutional norm, or something that should not be normalized at all.
- An unclear standard and a standard you failed to meet are different problems.
- A few early questions can make tacit expectations explicit before they become corrections.
- When feedback conflicts, look for whether supervisors are judging different parts of the same task.
- Decide what should travel with you: a real skill, a local preference, or neither.

PART III

Learning While Being Watched

Much of clinical learning happens in front of other people. The people observing you may also be teaching you, supervising your work, evaluating your performance, and deciding how much responsibility to entrust to you.

Learning therefore happens while developing skills are visible to people whose judgments may have consequences. That changes the context in which ordinary learning problems occur.

A question you could answer privately may feel different when an attending asks it on rounds. A decision may carry additional meaning when you know your resident is also judging what responsibility to give you next.

You may hesitate before asking for help because you are trying to determine whether the question is one you should already be able to answer. You may also be given more responsibility before that responsibility feels familiar, even when the supervision around you remains appropriate.

Part III examines what happens when learning, supervision, evaluation, and increasing responsibility occur at the same time. The central question is: **What changes when the people teaching you also supervise, evaluate, and decide how much responsibility to entrust to you?**

Chapter 7 begins with responsibility. It asks what happens when the responsibility you are given changes faster than your subjective familiarity with performing that part of the role.

Chapter 8 turns to help-seeking. It examines why recognizing that you need another person and actually involving that person are separate problems, especially within hierarchy.

Chapter 9 focuses on uncertainty itself. It asks what remains unresolved when "I don't know" appears and whether the next move is more knowledge, more information, clarification, supervision, escalation, continued reasoning, or action despite uncertainty.

The social conditions of training belong in the analysis because they affect what learners are being asked to do and under what conditions they are trying to do it. They do not explain every difficult performance, and they should not be used to make genuine gaps disappear.

The aim is greater accuracy about the task, the responsibility surrounding it, and the conditions under which the learner is trying to perform it. Part III adds the social environment to the differential without making it the default explanation.

CHAPTER SEVEN

When They Think You're Ready Before You Do

Your resident hands you the phone number for the consultant and says, "Why don't you make the call?" You have listened to consult calls before, and you know why the team is calling. You can summarize the patient and explain the clinical question, but you still expected your resident to make this one.

You look at the number, then back at her. She has already turned toward the computer because, from her perspective, the next step appears settled. You make the call. It goes reasonably well, although you spend most of it acutely aware that you are the person speaking on behalf of the team.

Afterward, your resident says, "Great. Let me know what they recommend." Nothing dramatic has happened. You have simply crossed one of the small thresholds that clinical training is full of: someone allowed you to do more of the work, while your own familiarity with being the person who does it has not necessarily changed at the same pace.

Two Clocks

It can help to imagine Two Clocks that do not always move together. The **responsibility clock** tracks what the role currently asks you to do and what supervisors are willing to entrust you to do under particular conditions. The **familiarity clock** tracks how established carrying that responsibility feels to you. For this book, treat those clocks as two pieces of information that may not move together. The Two Clocks are a practical synthesis, not an established developmental model.

You may be trusted to see a patient with less direct prompting before doing so feels ordinary. You may be expected to propose a plan while still experiencing your own plans as provisional thoughts that probably belong inside your head until someone asks.

You may be asked to make the consult call, perform part of a procedure, communicate an update, or take the lead on a task that recently belonged more visibly to someone above you. Responsibility can change in a single sentence, while familiarity may change more gradually.

This difference can produce a troubling interpretation: *If I were really ready, shouldn't this feel more natural?* Feeling unfamiliar does not by itself answer that question. You may simply have had fewer opportunities to carry this part of the role.

That does not establish that every increase in responsibility is appropriate. It tells you that **feeling unfamiliar with a role and being unprepared for every part of that role are different questions.**

Entrustment Is More Specific Than "They Think I'm Ready"

It is tempting to describe increasing responsibility by saying that other people think you are ready. That language is too broad.

Entrustment is more specific than a global judgment that a learner is "ready." In entrustment-based education, judgments concern whether a learner can be trusted with particular professional activities at an appropriate level of supervision (ten Cate, 2013). Being entrusted with one activity therefore does not mean that a supervisor believes you can perform that activity without supervision in every setting.

Consider the consult call. Your resident may trust you to make the initial call while remaining available if something unexpected arises and reviewing the consultant's recommendation afterward. That is different from deciding that you no longer need supervision around consultation decisions.

The same distinction applies when a resident asks you to see a new patient first. The invitation may mean *I think you can begin this task and bring me what you find* rather than *I think you should be able to manage this patient without me.*

Students can turn bounded entrustment into a much larger internal standard: *They let me do this, so I should no longer need help with it.* That conclusion does not necessarily follow.

A more useful question is: **What part of this task am I being trusted to do, and where does supervision still belong?** The responsibility becomes easier to interpret once its boundaries are visible.

Responsibility Can Change Before Familiarity Does

Think about the first time you were expected to propose a plan rather than report what had already been decided. You may have understood the patient well enough to generate reasonable options, while saying "I think we should..." still felt different from thinking those options privately.

Making the recommendation visible is the responsibility half — another person can now evaluate it, question it, or act on it. The familiarity half lags behind simply because you have had fewer experiences occupying the position of the person who recommends rather than reports.

The practical point does not require a theory of identity. You may become able to carry a responsibility before carrying it feels ordinary.

That difference may narrow with experience. The first consult call can feel consequential, while later calls may become another part of the day. The first time you offer a plan before anyone asks may feel presumptuous; later, arriving without a plan may feel incomplete.

The responsibility did not become appropriate because it eventually felt familiar. Familiarity and appropriateness are separate questions, which is why the supervision surrounding the task still matters.

What Does the Role Actually Require Today?

When responsibility increases, you can begin comparing yourself with an imagined version of the person who should occupy the role:

- *A fourth-year should know this.*
- *If they trust me with this patient, I shouldn't need to ask.*
- *If I'm ready for residency, this shouldn't feel difficult.*

These statements combine two questions that should remain separate. One concerns what your current role actually requires. The other concerns what you think someone in that role should already know, do, or feel like.

Ask first: **What am I actually expected to do at my current level?** Then ask: **Which parts am I expected to carry myself, and where is supervision still appropriate?**

Those questions move the standard back toward behavior. You may discover that your job is to gather the information, form an initial assessment, propose a plan, and bring relevant uncertainty to your resident before action is taken.

That is much more usable than *act like a fourth-year*. It also prevents subjective familiarity from becoming the standard for whether you are allowed to participate.

They Can Be Wrong Too

Clinical training is relational. You do not decide entirely by yourself when to take on more responsibility because supervisors also observe your work and decide what they are willing to let you do.

Those decisions can create opportunities to participate in work you might not yet have volunteered to do on your own. A supervisor's decision to give you more responsibility is one piece of evidence about how that supervisor is judging your performance in that task and context.

If several supervisors who know your work begin allowing you to carry more of a particular task with less prompting, that change tells you something about how they are assessing your performance in those situations. It is still not an infallible verdict about your overall readiness.

This is where Part II remains useful. Ask what was actually observed, what standard was being applied, and how much evidence the judgment can carry.

You do not need to replace *I don't feel ready* with *They think I'm ready, so I must be.* Instead ask: **What evidence led**

to this level of responsibility, and what does this particular responsibility actually require from me?

Use the Responsibility as Information

Suppose your resident asks you to lead the discussion of the assessment and plan for your patients tomorrow. Your first reaction is that you are not ready. Instead of trying to manufacture confidence, make the responsibility more specific.

What will you actually need to do? You will need to identify the active problems, decide what you think is happening, propose reasonable next steps, and make relevant uncertainty visible when it affects the plan.

Then identify where supervision remains. Your resident and attending are still present, and your plan will still be discussed before the team acts on decisions outside the responsibility you have been given.

That turns a role-level fear into a task you can prepare for. You might review each patient and write down:

- **What is the main problem today?**
- **What do I think we should do?**
- **What am I uncertain enough about that I need to check?**

Then participate at the level you have actually been asked to participate. Let the experience generate more evidence about what you can do and where you still need support.

The goal is not to feel ready before acting. It is to understand the responsibility well enough to participate within its boundaries appropriately.

Lagging Is Not a Defect

You may notice that your external role changes faster than your internal language. People begin asking what you think rather than what you found. A nurse asks you a question about your patient before you have adjusted to being someone who might know the answer.

A junior student asks you how something works, and your first thought is that they should probably find someone more qualified. Then you realize that you actually can answer the question.

You do not need a name for this experience. Responsibility, participation, recognition from other people, and your own familiarity with the role may not change at the same pace. That is enough to tell you what to examine when the role feels ahead of you.

Ask whether you can perform the behaviors the role currently requires. Ask what evidence supervisors appear to be using when they give you responsibility, and identify which parts of the role remain unfamiliar because you have had limited experience carrying them.

Then keep watching the trajectory. If the task becomes more familiar with appropriate participation and supervision, that pattern gives you additional information about what was new and what still requires support.

When Feeling Unready Contains Useful Information

The familiarity clock should not be dismissed simply because responsibility has advanced. Sometimes *I don't feel ready* contains information worth investigating: you may never have performed a particular task, remain unclear about an important part of it, or not understand what your supervisor expects you to handle yourself.

Translate the feeling into a specific uncertainty. Instead of "I'm not ready to do this," you might say, "I can take the history and form an initial assessment, but I haven't done this procedure before and need you to walk me through the setup."

Instead of "I don't think I can handle this patient," you might say, "I can see the patient and start the evaluation, but I'm unsure which findings would require me to call you immediately." The second versions give another person something they can respond to. They also help distinguish general unfamiliarity from a specific knowledge, experience, or supervision need.

This is where the Two Clocks become useful rather than reassuring. The familiarity clock tells you where the role still feels new, while the responsibility clock tells you what you are currently being asked to do. The task is to identify where the difference calls for experience and where it calls for clarification, preparation, or additional supervision.

Being Trusted Is Not a Test

Increasing responsibility can create a risky misunderstanding: if someone has entrusted you with the task, asking for help means you have failed the test. That conclusion treats independence as unsupported performance. In one study of prospective entrustment decisions across undergraduate and graduate medical education, faculty described knowing one's limits and seeking help as foundational to entrustment rather than evidence against it (Schumacher et al., 2022).

Greater learner independence can coexist with ongoing clinical oversight. Supervisors may monitor trainee work routinely, respond when concerns arise, or conduct some oversight without the trainee being directly aware of it (Kennedy et al., 2007). Being given more to do does not mean that appropriate supervision should disappear.

You may be expected to attempt more of the task yourself while still being expected to involve another person when the situation exceeds your role, knowledge, experience, or authority. **Responsibility before confidence is not the same thing as responsibility without appropriate supervision.**

Chapter 8 will examine why recognizing that you need help and actually involving another person can become complicated under hierarchy and evaluation. Here, the important point is that increasing responsibility does not eliminate the legitimacy or necessity of appropriate supervision.

Let the Clocks Move

You will not always feel like the person other people are beginning to treat you as. That experience does not automatically mean they have overestimated you, and it does not automatically mean their judgment is correct.

Ask what responsibility has actually changed. Identify the task, what part of it you are being asked to carry, and the supervision that remains available. Then separate those questions from familiarity: notice which parts of the role you can already perform and which remain unfamiliar because you have done them only a few times.

Let repeated experience provide more evidence. A task that feels consequential today may become more familiar after you have performed it with appropriate supervision, received feedback, and learned where its boundaries are. If the responsibility exceeds what you can safely manage with the supervision available, that requires a different response from simply wishing the role felt more familiar.

The Two Clocks do not need to move together. **Being trusted with more responsibility is not the same as feeling familiar with that responsibility.** What matters is whether the responsibility is appropriately bounded, whether supervision still fits the task, and whether you can identify what support you still need.

Stabilizing Shift

When responsibility increases faster than it feels familiar, that gap is not evidence you do not belong — it is the ordinary lag between the responsibility clock and the familiarity clock.

Options Menu

- **Name what you are actually being trusted to do.** Entrustment is usually bounded to a specific task, not a global verdict on your readiness.
- **Translate the feeling into a specific uncertainty.** Instead of "I'm not ready," try "I don't yet know how to manage rapid dosing changes without more support."
- **Use the new responsibility as information.** Identify what you will actually need to do and where supervision still applies, rather than waiting to feel ready.
- **Remember supervisors can be wrong too.** If several people who know your work converge on trusting you with more, that is real evidence — but any one person's judgment can still miss something.

Common Trap

Treating "they think I'm ready" and "I feel ready" as though they must match before you can act. Waiting for the internal clock to catch up to the external one can stall you well past the point where you are actually capable of the task.

A calmer alternative: ask what the role requires today, then act at the level you have actually been asked to participate.

Recap

What to remember when stressed:

- The responsibility clock and the familiarity clock do not have to move together.
- Entrustment is usually specific to a task, not a global judgment about your readiness.
- Translate "I'm not ready" into a specific, checkable uncertainty.
- Supervisors' trust is evidence, but supervisors can still be wrong.
- Lagging behind your new responsibility is not a defect — watch whether the gap narrows with experience.

CHAPTER EIGHT

Why Didn't You Just Ask?

The potassium comes back higher than you expected. You look at the result again, then at the rest of the morning labs. You are not sure whether this is something your resident needs to know immediately or something you should understand better before interrupting her.

She is on the phone with a consultant. The team is already behind, and twenty minutes ago you asked her a question that, in retrospect, you probably could have answered yourself. You open the chart and start looking for the previous potassium. Maybe there is an obvious explanation, or perhaps you should check whether the sample was hemolyzed before saying anything.

A few minutes pass. Later, someone asks why you did not tell the team sooner. The question sounds simple: *Why didn't you just ask?*

From the outside, help-seeking can look like a single decision: you either asked or you did not. From inside the situation, several decisions may come before that one.

You had to recognize that you needed another person, understand how quickly that person needed to become involved, know whom to approach, decide how much you were expected to work through yourself, and judge whether the person was realistically available. You were also doing all of this inside a social environment where previous interactions may have taught you that questions are welcome, tolerated, inconvenient, embarrassing, or costly.

A grounded-theory study of clinical teaching teams found that trainees' decisions about requesting clinical support involved more than the clinical question itself. Supervisor availability and approachability, perceptions of their own skill and independence, evaluation, and concerns about professional credibility also entered the decision (Kennedy et al., 2009).

If help-seeking breaks down, *I should have asked* identifies the outcome. It does not yet tell you where the path to help broke down. For this book, it helps to locate that breakdown before deciding what the learner should have done differently.

Did I Recognize That I Needed Help?

The first problem can occur before help-seeking begins. You cannot ask for help you do not realize you need.

Imagine that you are seeing a patient whose blood pressure has fallen since the morning. You notice the number, but you do not yet understand its significance in the context of the patient's other findings. You continue gathering information because you think you are still solving the clinical problem. Only later do you realize that the change should have prompted earlier involvement from your supervisor.

That is different from recognizing immediately that something may be important and choosing not to tell anyone. The visible outcome may be identical, while the breakdown occurred in a different place.

This distinction matters because "ask for help sooner" may not address the first problem. If you did not recognize the significance of the finding, you may need more knowledge, more experience recognizing concerning patterns, or clearer guidance about situations that require immediate communication — Chapter 2's performance differential still applies. Telling yourself to be more willing to ask questions will not teach you which clinical changes should trigger one.

Did I Understand the Urgency?

You can recognize uncertainty without recognizing urgency. You know that you need your resident eventually; the unresolved question is whether *eventually* means after you review the chart, after rounds, or now.

This distinction matters because some uncertainty can remain unresolved while you gather more information. Other uncertainty needs to become visible before you have completed your reasoning.

Suppose you receive a result that seems concerning but you are unsure whether you are interpreting it correctly. You may feel pressure to understand the problem before bringing it to someone else.

In some lower-stakes situations, working through part of the question before involving someone else may give you an opportunity to practice your own reasoning. That does not make delayed involvement the right response when the information could require timely action.

In those situations, finishing your analysis may matter less than making the concern visible to someone with the appropriate responsibility. You do not need to know exactly what the result means before saying: "This value changed substantially from yesterday. I'm not sure how significant it is, and I wanted to make sure you saw it."

The statement makes your uncertainty explicit without requiring you to solve it first. One of the most important boundaries in this chapter is that **when patient safety is involved, you do not need certainty before making the concern visible.**

Did I Know Whom to Ask?

Sometimes you recognize the need and understand the urgency, but the route to help is unclear. Your resident is unavailable, the attending is in a procedure, and another resident is covering but does not know you or the patient.

You may know that someone needs to become involved without knowing who the appropriate person is. In a familiar environment, the escalation route may seem obvious, while a learner entering the system may still be discovering it.

This is partly a system problem. "Ask for help" is incomplete advice when the learner does not know where help is located.

The practical response is to clarify consequential escalation routes before you need them. Early in a clinical setting, you might ask who you should contact if your immediate supervisor is unavailable and something cannot wait.

You do not need a map of every possible contingency. You need enough information to know where to go when the ordinary route fails.

If a situation is urgent and your usual supervisor is inaccessible, use the appropriate available clinical or institutional escalation route. The exact route will vary across settings, which is why local supervision and escalation expectations need to be made clear.

Did I Know How Much I Was Expected to Handle Myself?

Chapter 7 established that greater responsibility can coexist with supervision. Here the question becomes more specific:

How far am I expected to take this problem before I involve someone else?

As you receive more responsibility, you have to distinguish problems you are expected to begin working through yourself from problems that require another person's involvement. Those boundaries are not always obvious.

You may worry that asking too early leaves too little room to develop your reasoning. You may also worry that asking too late will make it look as though you failed to recognize your limits.

Sometimes a supervisor can make the boundary explicit. You might ask: "For problems like this, would you like me to work through an initial plan and bring it to you, or tell you as soon as I recognize the issue?"

That question clarifies the expected relationship between your own reasoning and supervisory involvement. Increasing responsibility does not mean delaying help for as long as possible. It means learning which parts of the work you can appropriately carry and where another person's involvement belongs.

Was the Person Realistically Accessible?

Advice about help-seeking often assumes that the appropriate person is available at the moment you recognize the need. Clinical work does not always cooperate.

Your resident may be responding to another patient, speaking with a family, scrubbed into a procedure, or managing several urgent problems at once. You may have been told to ask questions freely while repeatedly encountering moments when asking feels practically difficult.

Accessibility is therefore different from willingness. You can be completely willing to ask and still have difficulty reaching the person you need.

When this happens, distinguish *I did not ask because I was afraid to ask* from *I tried to obtain help and could not access the appropriate person.* Those problems require different responses.

For recurring accessibility problems, clarify backup routes. Ask whom to contact when your usual supervisor cannot be reached and what kinds of concerns should bypass the ordinary workflow.

If the available supervision is consistently inadequate for the responsibility you have been given, the problem is larger than your help-seeking technique. **Responsibility requires a workable route to appropriate support.**

What Has This Environment Taught Me About Revealing Uncertainty?

Now consider a different situation. You know you need help, know whom to ask, and know that the person is available, but you still hesitate.

Perhaps the last time you asked a question, your resident responded, "You should know this by now." Maybe you have watched another student get mocked for asking something basic. Perhaps nothing explicitly hostile has happened, but your attending moves quickly, rarely invites questions, and seems irritated whenever the team slows down.

Research on psychological safety in medical education emphasizes that it is shaped by interpersonal and organizational conditions, not simply by a learner's willingness to speak. A 2023 scoping review found a developing but still limited medical-education evidence base examining psychological safety in relation to learning, well-being, and the learning environment (McClintock et al., 2023). **That does not mean every hesitation to ask for help is evidence of low psychological safety.**

You may hesitate because you have not recognized the need for help, do not know how urgent the problem is, do not know whom to ask, are uncertain about your responsibility boundary, cannot readily access the appropriate person, or anticipate a social cost for revealing uncertainty. Learners can also hesitate in otherwise supportive environments. You may fear looking incompetent, misjudge what you should already know, or simply dislike interrupting someone with more authority. The useful question is therefore specific: **What has this environment actually taught me about what happens when people reveal uncertainty or ask for help?**

Look for evidence. What happens when other learners ask questions, admit mistakes, disagree, or say they are unsure? Then separate what you have observed from what you fear might happen. Both can influence behavior, but they are different evidence.

Sometimes the hesitation belongs mostly to your interpretation of the situation. Sometimes the environment has repeatedly demonstrated that revealing uncertainty carries a social cost. Those situations require different responses: a clearer request may help with the first, while the second may require another person, another route, or support beyond the immediate interaction.

Make the Question Easier to Answer

When asking for help feels exposing, the request itself can become harder to formulate. You may bring so little information that the other person has to reconstruct the problem, or so much that the question disappears inside the explanation.

"I don't know what to do" leaves the supervisor to reconstruct the entire problem. A five-minute account of everything you have considered can hide the question you actually need answered.

A simple structure can make your reasoning and your need visible:

- Here is what I see.
- Here is what I think.
- Here is what I do not know.
- Here is what I need from you.

Suppose a patient's blood pressure has fallen and you are unsure what to do next:

"Her blood pressure is now 86/52, down from 112/70 this morning. She looks more tired, but I haven't found an obvious source of bleeding. I'm not sure how concerned we should be about the change, and I'd like you to see her with me."

You have not pretended to know more than you know, and you have not handed over the problem without showing what you noticed and how you are thinking. The structure can be shorter when the situation is urgent. Its purpose is clarity, not performance: you are telling another person what you see, what you currently think, where your reasoning reaches its limit, and what you need next.

Asking Too Early and Asking Too Late

There is a developmental tension here, but there is no single threshold that fits every task. If someone else routinely takes over before you have a chance to work through the problem, you may have fewer opportunities to practice your own reasoning.

Waiting too long creates a different problem. The task may exceed your role, require authority or expertise you do not have, or need more timely involvement.

The goal is therefore neither maximal independence nor maximal supervision. It is learning where your own reasoning can appropriately continue and where another person's involvement belongs.

That boundary changes with the task, the stakes, your current responsibility, and the supervision available. A changing clinical situation may need to become visible while you are still investigating it, which is why "just ask" is inadequate as a universal instruction.

When You Should Have Asked

The environment matters, but it cannot become an explanation that makes every missed escalation disappear. Sometimes the expectation was clear: you recognized that something was concerning, knew that your supervisor wanted to hear about it, had a reasonable way to reach them, and still decided to wait.

That deserves a direct response. Ask what led you to delay and what you need to change the next time the same situation occurs.

Perhaps you were trying to appear independent. Maybe you wanted to bring a complete answer instead of an unresolved concern, or you underestimated how much the timing mattered. Those are useful findings because they identify a specific decision that can change.

You do not need to turn the event into *I am unsafe* to take the event seriously. The same principle from earlier chapters applies: identify the breakdown accurately enough to choose a response that addresses it.

When "Just Ask" Is Not Enough

There are also environments where ordinary help-seeking does not work as it should. A learner may repeatedly be humiliated for appropriate questions, discouraged from escalating concerns, unable to reach necessary supervision, or pressured to perform beyond an appropriate level of responsibility.

In those situations, becoming more skillful at phrasing the request may not solve the underlying problem. The next move may involve another supervisor, a clerkship or program leader, an institutional reporting or support route, or another appropriate professional resource. The specific route will depend on the setting and the nature of the concern.

The boundary is especially clear when patient safety is involved. You do not need certainty before making the concern visible, and impression management should not take priority over appropriate escalation.

Students can work on recognizing when they need help and communicating that need clearly. They cannot guarantee that every environment will respond appropriately, and that distinction protects agency without assigning learners responsibility for conditions they do not control.

Where Did Help-Seeking Break Down?

After a moment when you wish you had asked sooner, "Why didn't I just ask?" is too blunt to teach you much. Work through the path instead:

- **Recognition:** Did I recognize that I needed help?
- **Urgency:** Did I understand how soon someone else needed to be involved?
- **Boundary:** Did I know how far I was expected to proceed myself?
- **Route:** Did I know whom to ask?
- **Access:** Was that person realistically available?
- **Social conditions:** What had this environment taught me might happen if I exposed uncertainty?

You do not need to conduct this analysis after every question you hesitate to ask. Use it when help-seeking repeatedly breaks down, when the stakes were meaningful, or when you cannot understand why you remained silent.

Then choose the response that fits the breakdown. You may need more knowledge to recognize concerning situations, clearer expectations about supervision, a backup route for escalation, practice making a concise request, or support in dealing with an environment where appropriate help-seeking has become costly.

The useful shift is from *I should be better at asking for help* to **Where did the path to help actually break down?** Once the breakdown is specific, the response can become more specific too.

That question also prepares you for Chapter 9. Before you can decide whether uncertainty requires another person, you first need to know what, exactly, remains unresolved.

Stabilizing Shift

When you wish you had asked sooner, resist the urge to just try harder next time — ask specifically where the help-seeking process broke down.

Options Menu

- **Use the four-part structure.** "Here is what I see. Here is what I think. Here is what I do not know. Here is what I need from you." It makes your reasoning visible, not just your uncertainty.
- **Clarify the boundary in advance.** Ask a supervisor directly: "For problems like this, would you like me to work through an initial plan first, or would you rather I check with you before I start?"
- **Identify the actual breakdown.** Was it recognition, urgency, knowing whom to ask, accessibility, or what this environment has taught you about revealing uncertainty?
- **Name environments that punish asking.** If the problem is genuinely social — not your own recognition or timing — becoming better at phrasing the question will not fix it.

Common Trap

Turning a single moment of delayed help-seeking into a global verdict — "I am unsafe" or "I should be better at asking for help." This protects a sense that the problem is fixable through personal effort alone, but it skips past the actual, more specific breakdown.

A calmer alternative: ask where in the process — recognition, urgency, boundary, route, access, or environment — things actually went wrong.

Recap

What to remember when stressed:

- Help-seeking is not one decision; it depends on recognition, urgency, knowing whom to ask, access, and what the environment has taught you.
- The four-part structure ("here is what I see...what I think...what I don't know...what I need") makes a request easier to answer.
- Asking too early and asking too late are both real risks — the right boundary changes with the task and your responsibility.
- If you delayed asking, find out what led you to wait before deciding what it means about you.
- When an environment genuinely punishes asking, the fix is the environment, not your phrasing.

CHAPTER NINE

What Kind of "I Don't Know" Is This?

You are asked what you want to do next for a patient, and your first thought is *I don't know*. The words are simple, but they can describe very different problems.

You may not know enough about the disease. You may know the relevant medicine while remaining uncertain which explanation best fits this particular patient.

You may know what needs to happen clinically but have never placed the order or performed the procedure. You may understand the decision but be unsure whether it is yours to make.

You may know what you want to do and have no idea how to make it happen in this hospital. Or you may be trying to interpret what another person expects from you before deciding what to say.

From inside the moment, all of these experiences can feel like uncertainty. *I don't know* is not specific enough to determine what you should do next, so the work of this chapter is to identify what, exactly, remains unresolved.

Locate What Remains Unresolved

Research in health care and medical education does not treat uncertainty as one undifferentiated state of "not knowing." Existing frameworks distinguish among different sources and domains of uncertainty and examine how context, subjective influences, and responses shape its experience (Han et al., 2011; Lee et al., 2021).

The distinctions in this chapter serve a different purpose. **They are practical places to look for what remains unresolved, not six established types of uncertainty.**

When *I don't know* appears, make the problem more specific. Is the missing piece information? Is the clinical situation itself unresolved? Do you not know how to perform the task? Are you unsure how far your responsibility extends? Are you trying to understand what another person expects? Or do you not yet know how the local system works?

You do not need to classify the uncertainty correctly. You need enough specificity to decide what question, information, person, or action might help next.

I Don't Know the Information

Your attending asks which organism most commonly causes a particular infection, and you cannot answer. You search your memory and find nothing reliable enough to use. The problem is relatively straightforward: you do not currently have the information available.

Sometimes you once knew the information and cannot retrieve it. Chapter 2 gives you a reason to distinguish missing knowledge from an access problem when that distinction changes what you should do next.

For the immediate uncertainty, however, the question is simpler: **Is there a knowable piece of information that I currently do not know?** If so, the response may be studying, looking something up through an appropriate source, or asking someone who knows.

Which response fits depends partly on the stakes and timing. A fact you need for next week's exam can wait for study, while information required for a decision affecting a patient now may need to be obtained now.

This kind of uncertainty does not need a more complicated interpretation. Sometimes *I don't know* means that there is something you need to know and do not yet know.

I Know the Information, but the Medicine Is Still Uncertain

Now imagine a different patient. You know the relevant physiology, understand the major diagnoses, and have gathered the information currently available. Several explanations remain plausible.

More studying may improve your reasoning, but it may not make the present case certain. The clinical situation itself may contain ambiguity that the available evidence cannot fully resolve.

Not all clinical uncertainty reflects missing knowledge in the learner. Uncertainty may also arise because the available information leaves diagnosis, prognosis, treatment, or another aspect of the clinical situation incompletely resolved (Han et al., 2011).

For the learner, the practical distinction matters. **If the missing piece is knowledge, seek the knowledge. If reasonable uncertainty remains after appropriate information gathering and reasoning, the task is different: decide what responsible action looks like while uncertainty remains.**

You may need to compare plausible explanations, identify what information would distinguish them, make a provisional decision, monitor what happens, and revise as new evidence arrives. The goal is not to feel certain; it is to reason appropriately with the uncertainty that remains.

I Don't Know How to Do This

Sometimes the medicine is clear and the action is unfamiliar. You understand why a procedure is indicated but have never performed it, or you know which test should be ordered but do not know the steps required to arrange it.

You may understand what needs to happen while lacking the procedural knowledge, technical skill, or local know-how required to make it happen. Ask: **Do I understand what needs to be done but lack the ability or experience to do it safely and reliably?**

If so, more reading may help only partially. You may need demonstration, supervised practice, a checklist, local instruction, or someone to perform part of the task with you.

The distinction matters because *I don't know how* can be misread as *I don't understand why*. Those are different gaps, and the response should target the part that remains unresolved.

I Don't Know Whether This Decision Belongs to Me

You recognize the problem and have an opinion about what should happen. What you do not know is whether you are supposed to act, recommend, ask permission, or simply make someone else aware.

Imagine noticing that a medication probably needs to be held. You understand the clinical reasoning but are unsure whether you should change the order, suggest the change to your resident, or wait for rounds.

The uncertainty is about the boundary of your responsibility rather than the medicine itself. Chapter 7 established that greater responsibility can coexist with supervision, so the useful question here is: **What part of this decision is mine, and where does another person's responsibility begin?**

If that boundary is unclear, clarify it. More studying will not necessarily resolve a question about who is expected to recommend, decide, act, or supervise.

I Don't Know What Another Person Expects or Intends

Your attending asks, "What else?" You cannot tell whether she thinks you missed the diagnosis, wants another item on the differential, or is simply asking you to continue reasoning aloud.

Your resident says, "Use your judgment," and you are unsure whether that means proceed independently or bring back a recommendation before acting. The unresolved question may be what another person expects, means, or intends you to do.

You may be able to infer some of it from context. Sometimes the more efficient response is clarification: "Do you want me to make the call and update you afterward, or check the plan with you first?"

That question turns an implied expectation into a more explicit one. Chapter 6 addressed the same problem from the perspective of standards; here, the point is simply that uncertainty about another person cannot always be resolved by doing more clinical reasoning. Sometimes you need information from the person whose expectation is unclear.

I Don't Know How the System Works

You know what needs to happen. You do not know how to make it happen here.

Who schedules the study? Which service performs the procedure? Does this consult require an order before you call? Who needs to approve the transfer?

These questions can feel embarrassingly basic because everyone around you seems to know the answers. Often, they know because they have spent more time in the system.

You may understand the clinical problem but still not know how this particular system turns the decision into action. That may require asking a resident, nurse, coordinator, clerk, pharmacist, or another person who understands the relevant workflow. The appropriate source of information depends on the question.

Unfamiliarity with the system can be easy to misread as a problem with your medical ability because the gap appears while you are trying to perform clinical work. The distinction from Chapter 1 remains useful: some competence travels, while some fluency is local.

Once you know what kind of information is missing, the response becomes simpler. Learn the relevant workflow rather than turning unfamiliarity with it into a verdict about your competence.

One "I Don't Know" Can Contain Several Problems

Real situations do not always fit neatly into one place. Suppose you are caring for a patient whose creatinine has increased after diuresis. You understand why the team is diuresing the patient but are unsure how the change in kidney function should alter the plan.

You might say:

"I understand why we're considering continued diuresis. I'm unsure how her kidney function changes that decision, and I'm also not sure which changes you want me to bring to you before rounds."

Now two unresolved questions are visible. One concerns the clinical decision, while the other concerns your responsibility for communicating it.

That is far more useful than *I don't know what to do*. You do not need to assign each uncertainty an official category; you need enough precision to see what information, person, or action might help.

Sometimes the response will have several parts. You may need to review the medicine, gather another piece of patient information, and discuss the decision with your supervisor.

Locating the uncertainty matters only if it changes what you do next.

What Would Reduce It?

When you notice yourself thinking *I don't know*, complete one sentence and then ask one question:

- **I am uncertain because __________.**
- **What would reduce this uncertainty appropriately?**

If you lack information, the answer may be studying or looking something up. If the clinical situation remains ambiguous, the answer may be gathering more evidence and reasoning provisionally.

If you do not know how to perform the task, you may need instruction or supervised practice. If the uncertainty concerns responsibility, clarify the supervisory boundary.

If you do not know what another person expects, ask. If the uncertainty concerns the local system, find someone who knows how that part of the system works.

The word *appropriately* matters because the goal is not always to eliminate uncertainty as quickly as possible. Sometimes obtaining more information would delay an action that needs to happen, and sometimes the uncertainty cannot be fully resolved with the information currently available. The response has to fit both the uncertainty and the situation.

Acting Before You're Sure

Some uncertainty cannot be resolved before action is required. A patient may change before the diagnostic picture is complete, or a decision may need to be made while several explanations remain plausible.

You may need to communicate a concern before you understand exactly what it means. Chapter 8 established the safety boundary: when patient safety is involved, you do not need certainty before making the concern visible.

The presence of uncertainty does not tell you to wait. It tells you to ask what can be clarified, what must remain provisional, what needs monitoring, and when someone else needs to be involved. Depending on the situation and your role, the response may include a provisional decision, additional supervision, escalation, monitoring, or an explicit plan for what information would cause you to change course.

Uncertainty does not remove the need to act when action is required. It changes what responsible action may look like, which is why *I need to be certain first* can become as problematic as pretending to have certainty you do not have.

Uncertainty Is Not Proof of Sophistication

There is a risk in a chapter like this. Once uncertainty is treated as an unavoidable part of medicine, uncertainty itself can begin to sound virtuous.

Uncertainty is neither proof of inadequacy nor proof of sophistication. Sometimes you are uncertain because the evidence genuinely permits more than one reasonable interpretation. Sometimes you are uncertain because you do not yet know something you are expected to know, and sometimes both are true.

At other times, you may need another person's judgment, while in a different situation you may have enough information and responsibility to make the decision appropriate to your role. **The feeling of uncertainty cannot distinguish those explanations for you.**

The existence of legitimate uncertainty in medicine does not make every instance of *I don't know* unavoidable or irreducible. Sometimes you need more knowledge, information, experience, clarification, or supervision. The useful question remains concrete: **What exactly is unresolved, and what would appropriately reduce, manage, or act within that uncertainty?**

Make "I Don't Know" More Precise

By this point in the book, the move should feel familiar: do not turn the feeling into the diagnosis. Get more specific.

- *I don't know the information.*
- *I understand the information, but the clinical answer remains uncertain.*
- *I don't know how to do this.*
- *I don't know whether this decision belongs to me.*
- *I don't know what this person expects.*
- *I don't know how this system works.*

These statements are not categories you need to memorize. They are prompts for locating the unresolved part of the situation — name what is unresolved, then ask what evidence, information, practice, clarification, supervision, or action fits that particular problem.

Sometimes the response will reduce the uncertainty. At other times, it will help you act appropriately while uncertainty remains.

Part III has been building toward this: you are learning while other people watch, supervise, evaluate, and decide how much responsibility to give you. Uncertainty remains part of that work.

"I don't know" identifies the presence of an unresolved problem, not its location. Before deciding what the uncertainty says about your competence, locate what remains unresolved and match the response to that problem.

Stabilizing Shift

When you notice yourself thinking "I don't know," ask what specifically is unresolved — information, the medicine itself, how to do something, whose decision it is, what someone expects, or how the system works.

Each needs a different response.

You can stop once the next step is clear. Reflection has done its job when it helps you act more wisely.

Options Menu

- **Complete the sentence twice.** "I am uncertain because ________." Then ask: "What would reduce this uncertainty appropriately?"
- **Separate a compound uncertainty.** A single "I don't know what to do" can contain both a clinical question and a system question — name each one separately.
- **Act before you are fully sure, when the situation requires it.** Communicating a concern does not require complete understanding first.
- **Check whether the uncertainty is legitimate.** Some uncertainty reflects a genuinely unresolved clinical question, not a gap in your knowledge.

Common Trap

Treating all uncertainty as the same problem, so that every "I don't know" gets the same response — usually more studying. This protects against the discomfort of not knowing what to do, but it wastes effort when the real gap is procedural, relational, or about the system, not informational.

A calmer alternative: locate the specific kind of "I don't know" before choosing how to resolve it.

Recap

What to remember when stressed:

- "I don't know" can mean at least six different things: missing information, unresolved medicine, an unfamiliar procedure, unclear ownership, unclear expectations, or an unfamiliar system.
- One moment of uncertainty can contain more than one of these at once.
- Ask what would reduce the uncertainty appropriately — the answer changes what you should actually do.
- Some situations require acting before uncertainty is fully resolved.
- Uncertainty is not proof of failure, and it is not proof of sophistication either — locate it, then respond to what you find.

PART IV

From Difficulty to a Useful Next Move

By this point, the book has given you several ways to investigate a difficult performance. You can ask what changed around you, where the performance broke down, what evidence you actually have, what standard was being applied, what responsibility you were carrying, what remained unresolved, and whether the conditions around learning affected what happened.

Those distinctions are useful only if they help you act. Part IV focuses on responding to difficulty without making every performance an ongoing investigation.

The central problem is timing. Some questions matter while the task is happening: Do I understand enough to continue? Does my current approach still fit? Do I need another person involved? Other questions can wait until afterward, when you have enough distance and evidence to examine what happened.

Part IV therefore asks a different set of questions: **Where should my attention be right now? How much investigation does this problem actually need? What response will produce useful information next?**

Chapter 10 begins with attention. It separates monitoring that remains connected to the task from self-surveillance that turns attention toward how you appear or what the performance seems to prove about you. The aim is not to stop monitoring yourself. It is to keep the questions that belong during the task connected to the work and leave larger verdicts for later.

Chapter 11 asks what else you are carrying. The same task can occur under different conditions: a new schedule, unfamiliar workflow, competing responsibilities, poor sleep, illness, or several changing demands at once. Those conditions do not explain every difficult performance, but they belong in the differential when the timing and pattern make them relevant.

Chapter 12 brings the method together. It shows how to use the smallest investigation that fits the problem: a brief differential when the next move is relatively clear and a deeper audit when the problem repeats, persists, carries meaningful stakes, or remains difficult to explain.

Part IV is therefore not an invitation to become more skilled at analyzing yourself continuously. It is about putting investigation where it can change what happens next. **Investigate enough to choose a useful next move, let the next performance give you more evidence, and then return your attention to the work.**

CHAPTER TEN

Don't Grade Yourself While You're Still Performing

You are halfway through presenting a patient when your attending looks down at the computer. You notice immediately. Maybe the presentation is too long. Maybe you already lost the main point, or perhaps she is simply entering an order and listening at the same time.

You keep talking, but part of your attention has shifted. You are now presenting the patient while also evaluating the presentation. Then you hear yourself hesitate and wonder whether the hesitation sounded uncertain, whether your resident noticed, and whether the attending's expression changed. A few seconds later, you realize that you have lost your place.

The problem is not that you monitored your performance at all. Clinical work requires monitoring. The useful distinction is between questions that remain connected to the task and questions that ask you to interpret yourself while the task is still unfolding.

What does the task require now? is different from **How am I doing, how am I looking, and what does this mean about me?**

Not All Self-Monitoring Is the Problem

Self-monitoring is necessary in medicine. You need to notice whether you understand enough to proceed, when you are reaching the limits of your knowledge, when your current approach no longer fits, and when another person needs to become involved.

Work on self-assessment in the health professions distinguishes broad judgments of overall competence from more situation-specific self-monitoring—awareness of whether one has the knowledge or skill needed for a particular problem. A 2023 scoping review of graduate medical education found that self-monitoring is highly dependent on time and context, while also finding that the literature remains heterogeneous and inconsistently defined (Eva & Regehr, 2005, 2011; Johnson et al., 2023). **For this book, the practical question is therefore not whether all self-monitoring is "good" or "bad," but what the monitoring is helping you do.**

For this chapter, three practical distinctions are enough:

- **Adaptive self-monitoring:** Do I know enough to proceed, or do I need information, supervision, or help?
- **Task monitoring:** Is what I am doing still fitting the task?
- **Self-surveillance:** How am I looking? How am I being judged? What does this performance seem to say about me?

Here, *self-surveillance* means attention directed toward how you appear, how you are being judged, or what the performance seems to say about you. I use the term descriptively rather than as the name of an established cognitive process, and I am not assuming that self-focused attention always impairs performance.

Adaptive self-monitoring and task monitoring stay connected to what the work requires. They can overlap, and the distinction between them matters less than whether the question keeps you connected to the patient, the task, the limits of what you know, or the need for support. Self-surveillance shifts attention from the work toward what the performance seems to say about you.

Checking, Not Judging

Suppose you are preparing to perform a task you have done several times before. Halfway through, you realize that you do not remember the next step reliably enough to continue.

The relevant question is not *Do I look incompetent if I stop?* It is *Do I know enough to proceed, or do I need another person involved?* That is the kind of situation-specific monitoring this chapter wants to preserve.

You may decide that you need your supervisor to talk you through the next step. You may pause to verify information or clarify what part of the task belongs to you. The monitoring remains connected to what the task requires and to the limits of what you can currently do without additional information or supervision.

The same applies to clinical reasoning. You may begin with a plausible interpretation and then realize that one important finding does not fit.

The useful thought is *My current explanation may not account for this finding.* That observation gives you a reason to reconsider the interpretation, gather more information, or involve someone else. The question remains about the patient and what the situation requires next, not about what noticing the mismatch proves about you.

Watching the Task

Now imagine that you are presenting a patient and notice that you have spent too long on the history without reaching the active problem. You shorten the next section and move to your assessment.

That is task monitoring. Your attention remains on the relationship between what you are doing and what the task requires: *Is this approach still helping me do what needs to be done?*

You can do the same thing on an exam. You notice that you have spent too long on one question, mark it, and move on because the remaining time matters. During chart review, you may realize that you are reading increasingly old notes without finding information relevant to today's problem, so you stop and return to the question you were trying to answer.

In each case, the monitoring remains connected to the work. It tells you something about whether the approach you are using still fits the task in front of you.

Watching Yourself Instead

Self-surveillance begins when the performance becomes partly a question about you:

- *Did that answer sound stupid?*
- *Why did I hesitate?*
- *Does my attending think I'm weak?*
- *Was that correction worse than the one the other student got?*
- *What kind of medical student still makes this mistake?*

These thoughts can feel responsible because they concern performance. The practical question is whether they give you information you can use in the task that is happening now.

Ask: **Does this thought help me understand the patient, respond to the question, adjust the task, or decide whether I need support right now?** If it does, use the information. If it is asking you to reach a broader conclusion about how you look or what the performance proves about you, that conclusion can usually wait. That is the central discipline of this chapter: **do not grade yourself while you are still performing.**

Someone Is Watching

Chapter 7 and Chapter 8 explained why clinical learning makes self-surveillance understandable. The people watching you may also evaluate you, supervise you, and decide how much responsibility to give you, so their judgments matter.

You therefore have good reasons to notice information coming from the environment. A supervisor's question, correction, or instruction may contain something you need to use immediately.

The problem is overextension. You hear "Can you say more about why you chose that?" and turn the question into *She thinks my reasoning is weak* before you have even answered it.

One task is explaining your reasoning. The other is deciding what the question says about your standing. The first belongs to the encounter; the second may deserve investigation later, when you have more evidence and the immediate task no longer needs your attention.

During Performance: Attend to the Task

The simplest rule in this chapter is also the most important: **during performance, attend to the task.** That does not mean ignoring useful signals from yourself, the patient, or the supervisor.

If you realize that you do not know enough to proceed, act on that realization. If your supervisor corrects you, use the correction. If the patient changes, update your thinking.

What you postpone is the broader judgment. You do not need to decide whether the mistake means you are behind while you are still trying to fix the mistake, and you do not need to interpret the attending's facial expression while she is asking you the next question.

Return to something concrete:

- What is the patient saying?
- What was I just asked?
- What information matters now?
- What is the next step?
- Do I need help before I continue?

These questions give you a place to return that remains connected to the work in front of you.

Use a Return Point

Telling yourself *stop thinking about yourself* may simply give you one more internal process to monitor. A Return Point is more concrete.

A Return Point is one task-relevant question you can use when you notice yourself moving toward self-surveillance:

- During a presentation: **What is the main clinical problem?**
- During a patient interview: **What did the patient just tell me?**
- During an exam: **What is this question actually asking me to distinguish?**
- During a procedure: **What is the next safe step?**

The Return Point should be small and immediately usable. **You are not trying to recover confidence. You are trying to rejoin the work.** Confidence may or may not return while the task is underway; you can still perform the next useful step.

After Ordinary Difficulty: Use a Brief Differential

Once the performance is over, some investigation may be useful. The introduction established an important rule: most hard moments need a useful next move, not a full investigation.

For ordinary difficulty, ask three short questions:

1. **What happened?**
2. **Where did the performance break down?**
3. **What should I do next?**

Keep the answers concrete. For example:

What happened?
I gave several possibilities but did not commit to one.

Where did it break down?
I had the information but could not prioritize it.

What should I do next?
On the next case, rank the top two diagnoses and state why one is more likely before discussing the rest.

That may be enough. You do not need to decide what the event says about your overall competence when you already have a specific explanation and a reasonable next test. Chapter 4's proportionality rule still applies: larger conclusions require more evidence. For an ordinary difficulty, the useful post-performance question is often simpler: **What would I change or test on the next attempt?**

After Repeated, High-Stakes, or Confusing Difficulty: Investigate More Deeply

Some problems deserve more than a three-question review. Use a Deeper Differential when the problem repeats, persists, carries meaningful stakes, or remains difficult to explain.

These are the moments when additional investigation may change the response. Perhaps several supervisors have identified the same weakness, a patient-safety concern occurred, or an intervention you expected to help has not changed the performance.

You may also need a deeper investigation when several plausible explanations remain alive. A performance problem may involve knowledge, prioritization, expectations, capacity, supervision, or more than one of them.

Chapter 12 will give you the full method for those situations. The important point here is timing: **do not use the full audit simply because an event felt bad. Use it when the problem needs more explanation than a brief differential can provide.** That keeps the method proportional to the problem instead of turning every uncomfortable event into a comprehensive review.

Reflection Should End Somewhere

Reflection is useful when it changes what you understand or what you will do. It has probably done enough when you can answer three questions:

- What happened?
- What is my current best explanation?
- What will I do differently or investigate next?

If you already have those answers and continue replaying the encounter, more analysis may no longer be serving the same function. You may find yourself asking questions that cannot be answered from the available evidence: *Did my resident lose confidence in me? Was that the moment they decided I am behind? Would a better student have handled that differently?*

Chapter 4 gives you a reason to recognize those as evidence problems. If you do not have information capable of answering them, additional analysis of the same event will not create that information.

When better evidence is needed, look for better evidence. When the useful lesson is already clear, allow the investigation to end and return to the next part of your work or life. The point of reviewing a difficult performance is to support a better next action, not to make every unanswered question about the event disappear.

Not Every Time

There is an obvious risk in a book built around careful interpretation. A conscientious reader can begin auditing every answer, presentation, pause, mistake, and awkward interaction until the Developmental Differential becomes a ritual performed after every uncomfortable moment.

That would defeat part of the book's purpose. Clinical days contain imperfections that do not all need investigation: missed details, weak answers, presentations that could be tighter, and misunderstandings about what another person wanted.

Some of those moments need a correction and another attempt. They do not all need a theory.

Use the brief differential when you need a next move and the Deeper Differential when the problem genuinely warrants it. Then let the next performance give you more information. The method is meant to reduce unnecessary self-interpretation, not provide a more sophisticated way to continue it.

What If the Moment Keeps Coming Back?

Sometimes you have already identified the lesson and the event still keeps replaying. Ask whether another pass is producing new information.

If you are noticing something you missed, clarifying what happened, or identifying a different response, the review may still be useful. If each replay produces the same conclusions, the process is no longer giving you new evidence.

At that point, more analysis is not automatically the next useful response. Depending on the situation, redirecting attention, talking with someone who has useful perspective, or seeking appropriate support may provide something the replay cannot.

If repeated self-analysis is consuming substantial time, interfering with sleep or functioning, or occurring alongside severe distress, use the support boundary established in the introduction. This book cannot determine the cause or severity of those experiences. The practical question remains functional: **Is reviewing the event still helping me learn**

or act, or is it only repeating information I already have?

What to Do on the Next Shift

Choose one situation in which you tend to start watching yourself perform. It might happen during presentations, when an attending asks follow-up questions, or when you are doing something while another person observes.

Before the next shift, pick one Return Point — reuse one of the examples above, or choose your own task-relevant question.

When self-surveillance appears, you do not need to argue with the thought. Return to the question.

Afterward, decide how much investigation the event deserves. If the difficulty was ordinary and the next move is clear, use the brief differential and move on. If it repeats, carries meaningful stakes, or remains difficult to explain, investigate more deeply.

The rhythm is simple:

- **During performance:** attend to the task.
- **After ordinary difficulty:** use a brief differential.
- **After repeated, high-stakes, or confusing difficulty:** investigate more deeply.

The purpose is not to think less carefully. It is to put different kinds of thinking where they are most useful.

Stay With the Work

You cannot prevent every self-conscious thought from appearing while you perform. Medical training gives those thoughts plenty of material, especially when the people observing you also supervise and evaluate you.

What you can do is decide which questions need an answer now. If the thought concerns safety, the limits of your knowledge, whether the current approach fits the task, or whether you need another person involved, use it.

If the thought is asking how you look, what someone thinks of you, or what one mistake proves about your competence or identity, postpone the verdict. That question may matter later, but the middle of the performance rarely gives you enough evidence to answer it well.

Stay with the patient, the question, the procedure, or the decision in front of you. Afterward, investigate only as deeply as the problem requires.

Do the work while you are doing the work. Investigate what it meant afterward—and only as deeply as the problem requires.

Stabilizing Shift

During a performance, ask what the task requires now — not how you are doing, how you look, or what someone thinks of you. Self-surveillance can wait until the task is over.

If this starts to become rumination, narrow the question: What changed, what evidence do I have, and what is one next move?

Options Menu

- **Use a Return Point.** Pick one task-relevant question in advance — "What is the main clinical problem?" — to come back to when self-surveillance begins.
- **Save the brief differential for after.** Once the task is over, ask what happened, where it broke down, and what to do next.
- **Match the depth of investigation to the problem.** Ordinary difficulty needs three questions; repeated, high-stakes, or confusing difficulty needs the fuller Deeper Differential.
- **Notice when reflection should stop.** If you already have your answers and you are still replaying the moment, more analysis is not adding information.

Common Trap

Treating every self-conscious thought during a task as something that needs resolving right then. This protects against the discomfort of an unanswered question about yourself, but it pulls attention away from the actual task while it is happening.

A calmer alternative: note the question, return to a task-relevant Return Point, and investigate the self-question afterward if it still matters.

Recap

What to remember when stressed:

- Not all self-monitoring is a problem — adaptive monitoring and task monitoring stay connected to the work; self-surveillance shifts attention to you.
- During performance, attend to the task; investigate what it meant afterward.
- Use a Return Point — one task-relevant question you can come back to.
- After ordinary difficulty, three questions are usually enough; save deeper investigation for repeated or high-stakes problems.
- Reflection should end somewhere — once you have an answer good enough to act on, stop.

CHAPTER ELEVEN

What Else Are You Carrying?

Something you usually handle well suddenly feels harder. You reread the same paragraph three times. A patient presentation that normally takes ten minutes to prepare takes twenty, and by midafternoon you are forgetting small things you usually catch.

The first explanation may be personal: *I am slipping. I should be able to handle this better.* Sometimes the performance really does reveal a knowledge or skill problem. Sometimes the conditions surrounding the performance changed enough that they belong in the explanation. That is the question for this chapter: **What conditions did I bring into this performance?**

Under What Conditions?

A performance never occurs in isolation. Sleep, workload, competing responsibilities, health, unfamiliar routines, emotional demands, and other conditions can change the circumstances in which a task is performed.

Their presence does not establish that they caused a particular result. It means they may belong in the investigation when the timing and pattern make them relevant, and they may change what response is worth testing.

A student who cannot explain acid-base physiology after adequate preparation has a different problem from a student who understands the physiology but is trying to use it during a week of disrupted sleep, a schedule change, and several competing demands. Both performances deserve attention, but they may not call for the same response.

A systematic review and meta-analysis of medical-student studies found modest associations between academic performance and sleep quality and daytime sleepiness, while sleep duration was not significantly associated with grades in the pooled analysis (Seoane et al., 2020). The practical implication here is modest: when performance changes during a period of substantial sleep disruption or fatigue, those conditions belong in the investigation. They do not automatically explain the result. The broader observational question is enough: **What changed in the conditions under which I was trying to perform?**

Capacity Is Evidence

Capacity is easy to moralize. When you have more energy, attention, or stamina, you may feel disciplined and capable. When those resources feel thin, you may decide that you are weak, inefficient, or failing to manage medical school correctly.

Neither conclusion follows automatically. Capacity is also easy to use as an excuse: *I was tired* can become a complete explanation for a poor performance before you have asked whether the underlying knowledge or skill was adequate.

Here, **capacity** is practical language for this book: a way to ask whether current demands, resources, and competing responsibilities are relevant to the performance you are trying to explain. It is not a validated construct, a fixed personal trait, or a measurable internal reserve. The useful position is in between: **treat capacity the way you would any other candidate explanation—something to weigh against the evidence, not something that resolves the question by itself.**

If several conditions changed at the same time, include them in the differential. Then ask whether the pattern of performance changes when those conditions change. **Capacity belongs in the differential as a hypothesis, not an escape hatch.**

What Else Changed?

Suppose a difficult week arrives during a new rotation. You are sleeping less, commuting farther, preparing for an exam, and learning a new workflow.

The task may look familiar. The conditions under which you are doing it are not. That does not prove that the surrounding demands caused the problem. It does tell you that *I suddenly became worse at this* is not the only explanation available.

Keep the description concrete. Instead of *I have too much going on*, ask what changed in ways you can observe.

Perhaps chart review takes longer because you are still learning the service. Maybe you are moving repeatedly between clinical work and exam preparation, or your schedule leaves less time between demanding days.

None of those conditions has to explain the entire difficulty. The point is to make them visible enough to ask whether they track with the performance.

Several adaptation demands can accumulate before earlier ones have become familiar. You may be learning a new role, workflow, schedule, set of expectations, or pattern of responsibility while also preparing for an exam or adapting to a significant change outside school. **Before interpreting one harder performance, notice how many things are changing around it.**

A Re-Entry Week

This distinction becomes especially useful when someone returns after time away. Imagine a student coming back after leave or another extended absence. The hospital may be familiar, the curriculum recognizable, and much of the medical knowledge still available.

At the same time, several parts of daily functioning may feel different from before: schedule, routine, local familiarity, retrieval, study rhythm, clinical workflow, expectations, health, or something else entirely. None of those changes should be assumed. They are possibilities to check before one difficult week becomes one global explanation.

A student may discover that the main problem is local fluency and routine. Another may find that a specific knowledge gap has emerged, while another may need support for something outside the ordinary learning process.

Re-entry does not come with a predetermined diagnosis. It is another situation where the Developmental Differential keeps the explanation open long enough to identify what actually changed.

Make Capacity Observable

Words such as *stressed*, *exhausted*, and *overwhelmed* can describe a real experience while still leaving you unsure what to do. They become more useful when you connect them to something observable.

Instead of stopping at *I'm stressed*, ask: **What changed in the work while I was under more strain?** Perhaps you are starting later, rereading without taking much in, losing track of unfinished tasks, switching between tasks more often, making fewer practice attempts, or skipping routines that usually help you stay organized.

Instead of stopping at *I'm exhausted*, ask where the change appears in the performance. These observations do not establish a mechanism or prove causation. They make the hypothesis specific enough to compare across situations.

I was tired is difficult to evaluate. *During weeks when my sleep is substantially disrupted, I notice that I lose track of pending tasks more often* gives you a pattern you can continue to examine without assuming what caused it.

That is the standard for this chapter. Capacity belongs in the analysis only when it helps make the performance more interpretable.

The Capacity Check

When a familiar task becomes unexpectedly difficult, use the **Capacity Check** as a short tool. Ask:

- **What am I adapting to right now?**
- **What changed outside this task?**
- **What demands are competing with it?**
- **What can I change?**
- **What requires support from someone else?**
- **What should not be solved by trying harder?**

The questions prevent two opposite errors. You do not want to ignore conditions that may be relevant to the work, and you do not want those conditions to become a universal explanation for every difficulty. The goal is to identify what belongs in the differential and what response becomes available once you see it.

What Am I Adapting To?

Start with changes that require active adjustment. A new rotation, schedule, commute, study demand, responsibility, or significant change outside school may be occurring while you are trying to maintain everything else.

You do not need to decide immediately whether one of these caused the problem. List what changed first, then ask whether the timing fits.

Did the difficulty begin as several adaptations accumulated, or was it present before those changes? If the difficulty predates the new demands, capacity may be less central than it first appeared. If it emerged alongside them, the changed conditions deserve a place in the differential.

What Is Competing With the Task?

Some conditions matter because other demands are present at the same time. You may be tracking unfinished patient tasks while trying to study, thinking about an exam while learning a new workflow, or carrying a significant personal concern into a day that already contains several responsibilities.

You do not need a cognitive mechanism to investigate the pattern. Ask: **What else am I trying to carry while I do this task?**

Then look for what changes. If one demand is reduced and the performance changes, that gives you information. If the same problem remains, reopen the differential.

What Can I Change?

Capacity problems can sound global until you look for something specific. You may be able to reduce the number of study resources you are using, simplify a morning routine, clarify who owns a task, move one optional commitment, or stop trying to repair several performance problems at once.

The response should fit the condition you identified. Adding another elaborate system to a week already containing too many moving parts may not address the problem you found.

Sometimes the next useful experiment is subtraction. If one unnecessary demand can be reduced, moved, postponed, delegated, or simplified, notice whether the performance changes.

Improvement does not prove that the removed demand caused the original problem. It does tell you that the conditions under which you were performing mattered enough to keep investigating.

At other times, the useful response is addition. You may need clearer priorities, more structured support, more direct supervision, or help with a task you cannot reasonably solve alone. The point is not that less is better. It is that **more effort should not become the default response before you understand what the problem requires.**

What Requires Support?

Some conditions cannot reasonably be solved through personal adjustment. If the problem involves unsafe workload, inadequate supervision, or working conditions that compromise learning or safety, better organization may not be enough. **A condition can be relevant to your performance without becoming your responsibility to fix.**

The same boundary applies when illness, severe distress, unsafe fatigue, or substantial or sustained functional impairment is present. Those situations require support appropriate to their nature and should not be reframed as capacity optimization.

A learner can recognize that inadequate supervision is affecting performance without being responsible for redesigning supervision. A student can recognize that a workload is unsafe without being responsible for making it safe. A person can recognize that illness is affecting functioning without treating illness as a productivity problem.

This chapter belongs in the Developmental Differential because conditions can change how a performance should be understood and what response makes sense. It does not turn every condition into something the learner is responsible for fixing.

Capacity Is Part of the Differential

This chapter could easily become a convenient explanation for every bad day. You were tired, busy, stressed, adapting, distracted, or carrying too much.

All of those things may be true, and you may still have missed something you were expected to know. **Capacity belongs in the Developmental Differential as a hypothesis, not an escape hatch.**

Ask what evidence makes the conditions relevant. Did the difficulty appear when several demands changed? Does the same problem occur when the surrounding conditions are more stable? Does the performance change when one of the conditions you identified changes?

If the difficulty becomes less pronounced, those conditions deserve more weight in the explanation. If the problem persists, reopen the differential and look again at knowledge, access, prioritization, execution, expectations, environment, supervision, or other plausible explanations.

More than one factor may still be contributing. You do not need to prove that capacity caused the entire problem. You need to know whether the conditions appear relevant enough that the response should include them.

Test the Capacity Hypothesis

Suppose you think current conditions are contributing to your recent performance. Ask what you would expect to see if that explanation were useful.

If unfamiliar routines are contributing, does the performance change as the workflow becomes familiar? If sleep or schedule disruption appears relevant, does the pattern change when those conditions change? If competing demands are part of the problem, does reducing one of them change what you can do?

If the same difficulty remains largely unchanged, capacity becomes a less complete explanation. That does not make the original hypothesis useless; several factors may have been contributing at once.

The result gives you new evidence. Use it to revise the working explanation and ask what else might explain the part of the problem that remains.

"I Was Tired" Becomes a Label

There is another trap here. You identify that you are sleeping poorly, carrying several demands, and struggling to keep up, then use that information to construct a different case against yourself: *I should have managed this better. Everyone else seems to handle the same schedule. I should be able to carry more than this.*

Some choices may deserve examination. That does not make capacity a moral score.

You can take responsibility for decisions that are actually yours without assuming that every condition was created by you. Training schedules, financial constraints, caregiving, health, learning environments, and institutional conditions may all be relevant to what you are carrying.

Comparison does not solve that question either. Another learner's visible performance does not tell you what conditions they are working under or what your own conditions should permit.

Keep both the learner and the environment in the analysis. Ask two different questions: **What can I reasonably change, ask for, stop doing, or investigate? What requires support, authority, accommodation, protection, or structural change beyond me?**

Sometimes the Next Useful Experiment Is Subtraction

When performance becomes harder, addition can be an automatic response: another resource, more questions, another study session, or a more elaborate schedule. Sometimes the additional plan becomes another demand without addressing the problem underneath it.

The Capacity Check should therefore allow subtraction. You might use fewer resources, reduce simultaneous goals, postpone something optional, or simplify what needs to happen this week.

That does not mean every difficult period calls for doing less. Some responsibilities cannot be removed, and genuine gaps may require additional learning or practice.

It means that more should not be the default response before you understand the problem. When an unnecessary demand appears relevant, reducing it can function as a test rather than as a failure of effort.

Know When This Is No Longer a Capacity Exercise

There is a firm boundary around this chapter. Illness, severe distress, unsafe fatigue, substantial or sustained functional impairment, and concerns about your own or a patient's safety should not be reframed as productivity or optimization problems.

If you are struggling to function in a way that is persistent, worsening, or affecting safety, seek appropriate professional, educational, supervisory, or institutional support. This book cannot determine the cause or severity of those problems or substitute for individualized evaluation.

The same boundary applies when working conditions themselves are unsafe. A learner should not be expected to manage dangerous fatigue, excessive demands, or inadequate supervision through better organization.

This matters because the language of capacity can sound deceptively manageable. **Some problems require support, protection, evaluation, or changes in conditions rather than a better personal strategy.**

The Capacity Check should help you recognize that boundary. It should not become another tool for remaining inside circumstances that require a different response.

Capacity Belongs in the Analysis

There will be weeks when you are doing familiar work under very different conditions. The same presentation may happen during a relatively stable week or while you are learning a new service and preparing for an exam.

Those differences do not erase the standard you need to meet. They may belong in the explanation of what happened while you were trying to meet it.

When a familiar task becomes unexpectedly difficult, ask what else changed around the performance. Then ask whether those conditions actually track with the pattern.

Capacity belongs in the analysis. It does not automatically explain the result.

Sometimes the next step will still be more learning or practice. Sometimes it will involve changing a condition, seeking support, or reducing an unnecessary demand.

The point remains the same as elsewhere in the book: **when performance changes, the focal task may not be the only thing that changed. Ask what else you are carrying, whether those conditions move with the performance, what you can reasonably modify, and what requires support or change beyond the learner.**

Stabilizing Shift

When a familiar task suddenly feels harder, ask what else changed around you — sleep, workload, competing responsibilities — before deciding something is wrong with your ability.

The goal is not endless self-analysis. The goal is better orientation.

Options Menu

- **Run the Capacity Check.** What am I adapting to right now? What is competing with this task? What can I change? What requires support from someone else?
- **Make the feeling observable.** Instead of "I'm exhausted," ask where the change actually shows up in your work — what you are skipping, losing track of, or doing more slowly.
- **Try subtraction before addition.** Reduce, postpone, or simplify one unnecessary demand and watch whether the performance changes.
- **Test it like any other hypothesis.** If the conditions are really contributing, the pattern should change when the conditions change. If it does not, look elsewhere.

Common Trap

Letting capacity explain everything — or refusing to let it explain anything. Both moves skip the actual evidence.

A calmer alternative: ask whether the difficulty tracks with the conditions you identified, not just whether the explanation feels comfortable or uncomfortable.

Recap

What to remember when stressed:

- A performance never happens in isolation — sleep, workload, and competing demands can belong in the explanation without automatically causing the result.
- Capacity is a candidate explanation to weigh against evidence, not a moral verdict or an automatic excuse.
- Use the Capacity Check: what you are adapting to, what is competing, what you can change, and what requires support.
- Try subtraction before adding more — sometimes the next useful experiment is doing less, not more.
- Illness, unsafe fatigue, and unsafe conditions are not capacity-optimization problems — they need real support, not better organization.

If you are testing whether an existing remediation or recovery plan is realistic given your life right now, *When Things Don't Go As Planned* goes further into that question.

CHAPTER TWELVE

What Changed? Build the Differential

Something happened, and you need to decide what to do next. Maybe the problem is obvious enough to act on immediately: you missed a question because you did not know the material, so you identify the gap and learn it.

Other problems are harder to interpret. A presentation goes badly even though you prepared. Feedback conflicts, or the same weakness keeps appearing after you thought you had addressed it. Several things changed at once, and you cannot tell which of them matters.

This is where the **Developmental Differential** becomes useful. It is this book's practical method for investigating a difficult performance before deciding what it means.

The goal is not to explain every variable that might have contributed. It is to identify enough of the problem to choose a response that fits and then learn from what happens next.

The 60-Second Differential

Most difficult moments do not need a deeper investigation. When the problem is ordinary and a useful next move becomes clear quickly, ask three questions:

1. **What happened?**
2. **Where did the performance break down?**
3. **What should I do next?**

Keep the answers concrete. Suppose you gave several possible diagnoses but never identified which one you favored. You may decide that the problem was prioritization rather than missing knowledge, and your next move may be to rank your leading diagnoses before the next presentation and state what distinguishes the first from the second.

If that gives you a useful next step, the brief differential has done enough. Let the next attempt give you more information rather than continuing to expand the analysis.

When to Use the Deeper Differential

Use the **Deeper Differential** when the problem repeats, persists, carries meaningful stakes, the evidence conflicts, or a well-matched response has not changed the pattern. It can also help when several explanations remain plausible and the 60-Second Differential does not tell you enough.

You do not need to revisit every concept in this book each time. The Deeper Differential follows one sequence and brings in earlier distinctions only when they help answer the question in front of you.

1. What Happened?

Describe the finding before deciding why it happened. *I am failing surgery* is too large, while *My presentations remain too long three weeks into the rotation, and two supervisors have told me that the main clinical problem is difficult to identify* gives you something you can investigate.

Then identify the interpretation that arrived with it. Perhaps it was *I should be better at this by now* or *I am bad at clinical medicine.*

Keep both visible. The first describes what happened; the second describes what you decided it meant. Neither one identifies the explanation by itself.

2. What Did I Decide It Meant?

Separate the event from the conclusion before expanding the investigation. Ask how far the interpretation reaches beyond what you actually observed.

A specific performance problem may deserve attention without supporting a broader verdict about competence. Chapter 4's proportionality rule still applies: **the farther a conclusion reaches beyond the event, the more evidence it should require.**

3. What Changed?

Now ask what changed around or within the performance. Did the environment change? Did the task retain the same name while requiring a different behavior? Did the standard change, or was an expectation still being learned?

Responsibility, supervision, access to help, local workflow, competing demands, and the conditions you brought into the task may also belong here. You do not need to assume that any of them explains the problem; identify what changed before deciding how much weight it deserves.

If nothing relevant changed, that is useful too. The question is not designed to produce a contextual explanation. It is designed to keep you from overlooking one.

4. Where Did the Performance Break Down?

Return to the practical distinctions from Chapter 2 when they fit:

- **Knowledge:** Did I understand enough?
- **Access:** Could I bring forward what I knew when I needed it?
- **Prioritization:** Could I decide what mattered most?
- **Execution:** Could I produce the performance reliably?
- **Environment:** Did something around the task interfere with what I was trying to do?

Do not force the problem into one category. Several may remain plausible, and another part of the book may provide a better explanation altogether. The purpose is simply to move closer to the point where the visible performance became difficult.

5. What Other Explanations Remain Plausible?

Keep two or three reasonable alternatives open long enough to compare them. A presentation that looks disorganized might reflect prioritization, execution, an unclear standard, a changed task, unfamiliar workflow, or more than one of those at once. This is where earlier chapters become useful without becoming a checklist. Ask only the questions that fit the event:

- Was the task asking something new?
- Was the standard clear?
- What did the feedback actually describe?
- Was the responsibility appropriately bounded?
- Did I know when and how to obtain help?
- What, exactly, remained uncertain?
- Did changed conditions belong in the pattern?
- Did self-surveillance become part of the event?

You are not trying to produce the longest differential. You are trying to prevent the first explanation from winning before you have compared it with plausible alternatives.

6. What Evidence Supports or Weakens Each Explanation?

Look at what you actually know. A knowledge explanation becomes more plausible if you still cannot explain the material later with time to think. An access explanation becomes more plausible if you can explain the material accurately later but repeatedly fail to bring it forward when the task requires it.

A standard problem becomes more plausible if expectations were unclear or inconsistent. A capacity explanation deserves more weight if the difficulty tracks with changed conditions and becomes less pronounced when those conditions change.

Feedback matters most when you can recover the observation underneath it. When repeated, reasonably specific observations continue to point toward the same problem, let that pattern change the working hypothesis rather than explaining each observation away separately.

Evidence can also weaken an explanation. If the task remains difficult after the condition you thought mattered has changed, that explanation may be incomplete. If you clarify the standard and the same performance problem remains, look elsewhere.

Broader Conclusions Come Last

Only after examining the event and the evidence should you ask whether the difficulty supports a broader conclusion about competence. **The farther a conclusion reaches beyond the event, the more evidence it should require.**

I omitted an important finding is a conclusion about one performance. *I repeatedly struggle to identify the important finding in complex cases* describes a pattern. *I am bad at clinical medicine* reaches much farther.

Sometimes the broader concern will survive the investigation. A persistent pattern across settings and repeated observations may support the conclusion that a broader area of competence needs attention.

The differential must remain capable of reaching that answer. Otherwise, it becomes reassurance disguised as analysis.

7. What Is My Current Working Hypothesis?

After considering the plausible explanations, stop generating possibilities. Choose the one or two that currently have the strongest support.

Suppose the problem is repeated disorganization during complex patient presentations. Your leading explanation might be prioritization, execution, or some combination of the two.

The evidence for prioritization might be that you struggle to decide what deserves emphasis even when preparing alone. The evidence for execution might be that you can identify the right hierarchy on paper but lose it during the live presentation.

You do not need to decide that one explanation is exclusively correct. **A working hypothesis only needs to be specific enough to guide the next useful response.**

8. What Response Fits?

Before choosing what to do, ask: **What would I expect to change if this explanation were useful?**

If prioritization is central, help identifying discriminating information might make the organization clearer. If execution is central, practice with direct observation might make the live performance more reliable.

If an unclear standard is central, clarification should change what you do. If changed conditions appear relevant, changing one of those conditions may change some part of the pattern.

You are not making a formal prediction about a controlled experiment. You are asking what information the next attempt could reasonably provide.

An explanation earns its place by telling you what evidence to look for next. The Developmental Differential is a practical synthesis of the distinctions

developed throughout this book, not a validated assessment model or a claim that these explanations exhaust every cause of difficulty.

9. Choose the Smallest Useful Response

Do not end the differential with ten findings and a ten-item self-improvement plan. Choose the smallest response—or small set of linked responses—that fits the leading explanation and gives you useful information about what happens next.

That response might include:

- targeted study
- retrieval practice
- help with prioritization
- coached performance
- clarification of expectations
- specific feedback
- appropriate supervision
- a change in conditions
- support
- escalation
- further assessment

Sometimes two responses belong together. You may need to review a knowledge gap and ask for direct feedback, or clarify a supervision boundary while also involving another person now.

The response should stay proportional to the problem. You are not trying to fix everything at once; you are choosing a response that fits the problem you currently have.

10. What Happened Next?

After the response, look again. Did the performance change, and if so, which part changed? Did the problem remain largely unchanged, or did something else become visible once the first problem improved?

Ask one more question: **What happened afterward that should change how much weight I give this explanation?**

This is the step that keeps the method provisional. **Without reassessment, a plausible explanation can become a permanent story.**

A working hypothesis should remain provisional enough to change when the next performance gives you different evidence. Sometimes your first explanation will survive; sometimes it will lose weight, and sometimes the next performance will show that several explanations were operating together.

Getting the first explanation wrong does not make the investigation useless. The goal was never to defend the first explanation; it was to move closer to the problem.

The Differential Must Be Allowed to Disappoint You

There is one final guardrail. A developmental framework can become sophisticated reassurance if every explanation eventually leads to the same conclusion: *the problem was understandable, so nothing is wrong.*

That cannot be how this method works. The differential must remain capable of producing an answer you did not want.

You may discover that you do not know something well enough yet, that a skill remains unreliable after appropriate practice, or that repeated observations continue to identify the same problem. The response you tried may not have changed it.

Those findings deserve attention because they make the problem more specific. The same discipline works in the other direction. You may discover that the standard was unclear, the feedback was not grounded in enough observation, the supervision was inadequate, or the conditions around the learner were part of the problem. **Accuracy has to work both ways.**

The purpose of the differential is not to reach the most reassuring explanation. It is to reach the explanation that currently fits the evidence best and remain willing to revise it.

Use the Smallest Tool That Works

Use whichever tool fits the problem: the **60-Second Differential** for ordinary difficulty, the full **Deeper Differential** when the problem repeats, persists, or resists a first response. Either way, stop investigating once you have a next move, and let what happens give you more evidence. The Developmental Differential is meant to improve action, not turn training into continuous self-investigation.

Its underlying sequence is simple:

1. **Event**
2. **Interpretation**
3. **Plausible explanations**
4. **Evidence**
5. **Working hypothesis**
6. **Response**
7. **Reassessment**

Start with what happened, not what you fear it means. Keep enough explanations open to examine the evidence, then choose a working hypothesis specific enough to guide a useful response.

Let the next performance change your mind when it gives you different information. Broader conclusions can wait until the evidence is broad enough to support them.

That is the method the book has been building toward. **The goal is not to decide quickly whether you are the**

problem. It is to find out what the problem is, what the evidence supports, and what useful move comes next.

Stabilizing Shift

Most difficult moments only need the 60-Second Differential: what happened, where did the performance break down, what should I do next.

Save the full ten-step Deeper Differential for problems that repeat, persist, carry real stakes, or resist a first response.

Do not turn this tool into another performance you have to master.

Options Menu

- **Run the 60-Second Differential first.** What happened? Where did it break down? What should I do next? If that gives you a usable next step, stop there.
- **Use the Deeper Differential's ten steps only when needed.** Finding, interpretation, what changed, where it broke down, plausible explanations, evidence, working hypothesis, response, and reassessment — in that order.
- **Choose the smallest response that fits.** One or two targeted changes usually beat a ten-item self-improvement plan.
- **Let the result update the explanation.** A working hypothesis that survives the next performance gets more weight; one that does not gets revised, not defended.

Common Trap

Treating the Deeper Differential as a tool for reaching the most comfortable explanation, rather than the most accurate one. A framework built to protect you from a hasty verdict can just as easily become a more sophisticated way to avoid an uncomfortable one.

A calmer alternative: let the differential stay capable of producing an answer you did not want — accuracy has to work in both directions.

Recap

What to remember when stressed:

- Most difficult moments need the 60-Second Differential, not a full investigation: what happened, where did it break down, what next.
- The Deeper Differential is for problems that repeat, persist, carry real stakes, or have not responded to a first attempt.
- Separate the finding from the interpretation, then ask what changed, where it broke down, and what other explanations remain plausible.
- Weigh the evidence for and against each explanation before committing to a working hypothesis.

- Choose the smallest response that fits, then let what happens next update the explanation — the differential has to be allowed to disappoint you.

CONCLUSION

Getting Better at Being New

Medical training does not reliably give you long stretches of stability. Just when a place, task, or role begins to feel familiar, something changes and part of the work becomes effortful again.

You learn how one team works and then join another. You become comfortable presenting straightforward patients and then encounter cases that require more judgment, compression, or responsibility. You learn how to prepare for one kind of assessment, then find that the next one asks you to use what you know differently.

Progress can therefore have a repetitive quality: something becomes familiar, then the conditions change and part of the work becomes unfamiliar again. That return of effort does not tell you by itself whether you have lost ground, encountered a real gap, or reached a situation that requires something different from you.

The endpoint of this book was never permanent confidence or permanent fluency. Medicine will continue to contain situations in which your knowledge, experience, information, responsibility, or authority is limited. The more durable capability is **reorientation**: knowing how to find your bearings when a performance becomes harder to interpret.

Research on transitions in medical education describes changes in context, participation, relationships, and expectations as learners move into new clinical environments, while work on adaptive expertise examines the need to adapt when familiar approaches are insufficient for a new problem (Atherley et al., 2019; Teunissen & Westerman, 2011; Mylopoulos & Regehr, 2009; Mylopoulos & Woods, 2017). The practical idea of reorientation in this book is a synthesis of that recurring problem, not a developmental-stage model.

Reorientation

Reorientation begins when you notice that something familiar has become harder and resist deciding too quickly what that change means. You look for what changed, where the mismatch may be, and what evidence distinguishes among the explanations still available.

Sometimes the answer is a genuine gap. You do not know enough yet, a skill is not reliable enough, or repeated observations identify the same problem. The appropriate response may be more learning, practice, feedback, or supervision.

At other times, the performance is occurring inside changed conditions. The standard may be different, the workflow unfamiliar, the responsibility new, the supervision unclear, or several demands may have changed at once. Those conditions do not erase the standard you need to meet, but they may change what response fits the problem.

Then you act and look again. If the response changes the performance, that gives you new information. If it does not, the explanation has to remain open to revision. **Reorientation means that difficulty can send you back to investigation without sending you immediately to a verdict about yourself.**

What You Can Carry Forward

You do not need to carry every distinction in this book into every difficult moment. A few questions can travel farther:

- **What actually happened?**
- **What changed?**
- **Where did the performance become difficult?**
- **How much does the evidence reasonably support?**
- **What response fits, and what happens next?**

Other questions become useful when the situation requires them. You may need to clarify a standard, recover the observation underneath feedback, locate what remains unresolved, identify the boundary of your responsibility, or ask whether the conditions surrounding the task belong in the explanation.

The point is not to perform the Developmental Differential perfectly. It is to have more precise ways into a problem than *I am the problem*.

Difficulty Before Judgment

Difficult days will still produce real information — missed knowledge, answers that need correction, skills not yet reliable. When repeated, specific evidence keeps pointing toward the same problem, let it change the working hypothesis; the Developmental Differential should make a genuine gap clearer, not make it disappear. The same discipline runs the other way: sometimes the standard was unclear, the task changed, or conditions around the learner contributed to what happened — recognizing that does not erase your responsibility, and your responsibility does not make every condition reasonable.

Accuracy has to work both ways. You should be able to identify a real gap without turning it into a verdict about who you are, and you should be able to identify a problem in the conditions without assuming that every difficulty is yours to fix.

Getting Better at Being New

You will be new again. Medical training will keep changing the places, tasks, standards, responsibilities, and problems through which your competence has to be expressed. The point is not to eliminate that newness or make every difficult transition feel comfortable.

What can change is what you do when newness makes your performance harder to interpret. You can begin with the event instead of the verdict. You can keep more than one plausible explanation open, look for evidence, choose a response that fits, and let what happens next change your mind.

Sometimes you will discover something you need to learn. Sometimes you will need practice, feedback, clarification, supervision, support, or a change in the conditions around you. Sometimes the first explanation will be wrong, and the next performance will give you a better one.

None of that requires you to decide immediately what the difficulty says about you. **A hard performance can deserve attention before it deserves a verdict. Getting better at being new means knowing how to begin when the conditions change again. Before you decide you're the problem, find out what the problem is.**

APPENDIX

Common Sentences This Book Is Trying to Interrupt

This appendix is not meant to talk you out of every hard thought. Some hard thoughts contain important information. The point is to slow the moment when a sentence about difficulty becomes a sentence about who you are.

When one of these sentences appears, try translating it into questions that can be answered.

"I'm bad at this."

- **What happened?** What specific task, moment, skill, or interaction led to this conclusion?
- **What evidence do I have?** Was this based on one event, repeated observations, formal feedback, comparison, exhaustion, or fear?
- **What changed?** Did the task require a new level of integration, speed, judgment, communication, or independence?
- **Where did it break down?** Knowledge, organization, retrieval, prioritization, confidence, workflow, feedback, supervision, or environment?

- **What does this require next?** Practice, teaching, feedback, rest, strategy change, clarification, support, or intervention?

"I should be better by now."

- **What happened?** What expectation did I believe I should already be meeting?
- **What evidence do I have?** Who set that expectation? Is it explicit, assumed, developmental, comparative, or self-imposed?
- **What changed?** Did I advance into a setting where the definition of "better" changed?
- **Where did it break down?** Was I missing skill, context, repetition, feedback, opportunity, or time in the role?
- **What does this require next?** A clearer benchmark, targeted practice, a supervisor's perspective, or a more realistic developmental timeline?

"I just need to study more."

- **What happened?** What made me reach for more studying as the answer?
- **What evidence do I have?** Did the difficulty come from not knowing, not retrieving, not applying, not prioritizing, or not communicating?

- **What changed?** Has the task shifted from recognition to application, from facts to judgment, or from isolated concepts to patient care?
- **Where did it break down?** Content knowledge, clinical reasoning, presentation, time pressure, task-switching, uncertainty, or fatigue?
- **What does this require next?** More study may help. But it may need to be a different kind of study: retrieval, cases, explanation, practice questions, oral presentation, simulation, or feedback-guided review.

"They think I'm ready, so I shouldn't need help."

- **What happened?** Where did I need support, supervision, confirmation, or backup?
- **What evidence do I have?** Did someone actually say I should not need help, or did I infer that from being advanced?
- **What changed?** Has responsibility increased faster than familiarity?
- **Where did it break down?** Was the issue independence, role clarity, uncertainty, patient safety, confidence, or knowing when to escalate?
- **What does this require next?** Clarify what decisions you are expected to make alone, what should be checked, and when help is required. Appropriate supervision is not the opposite of competence.

"If I were competent, this wouldn't feel hard."

- **What happened?** What felt hard: the task, the pace, the ambiguity, the responsibility, the emotion, or the meaning you attached to it?
- **What evidence do I have?** Is the feeling of difficulty matched by observed performance, or is it mainly an internal signal?
- **What changed?** Did you move into a more complex environment where competent performance still feels effortful?
- **Where did it break down?** Was there an actual performance gap, or did the work feel unfamiliar, exposed, or high stakes?
- **What does this require next?** Treat the feeling as information, not a verdict. Look for external evidence, specific feedback, and one skill or condition that can be adjusted.

"I got feedback, so it must be true."

- **What happened?** What was the exact feedback?
- **What evidence do I have?** Was it specific, behavioral, repeated, observed directly, aligned with other feedback, and tied to expectations?

- **What changed?** Did the feedback come in a new environment with different norms, preferences, or hidden criteria?
- **Where did it break down?** Was the issue the performance itself, the interpretation of the performance, the delivery of the feedback, or a mismatch in expectations?
- **What does this require next?** Do not dismiss feedback because it hurts. Do not absorb it whole because it hurts. Translate it into observable behavior and ask what improvement would look like.

"I feel behind, so I must be behind."

- **What happened?** What triggered the feeling of being behind?
- **What evidence do I have?** Am I comparing myself to clear standards, selected peers, imagined expectations, or my own previous ease?
- **What changed?** Did I enter a new group, role, block, service, hospital, specialty, or level of responsibility?
- **Where did it break down?** Actual progress, perceived pace, visibility of others' work, feedback, belonging, or confidence?
- **What does this require next?** Find the real benchmark. Ask what is expected at this stage, what

would need attention, and what one next step would narrow the gap if a gap exists.

Before You Decide: A One-Page Differential

- **What happened?** Name the event without exaggerating it.
- **What did I decide it meant?** Write the conclusion your mind reached.
- **What changed?** Look for changes in task, environment, expectations, responsibility, feedback, or support.
- **Where did the performance break down?** Locate the problem as specifically as possible.
- **What evidence do I have?** Separate observation from assumption and pattern from single event.
- **What support may be needed?** Teaching, coaching, clinical care, disability support, or institutional help.
- **What is the smallest useful next move?** Choose one action that can produce more information or reduce the problem.
- **What would I watch afterward?** Notice whether the problem improves, repeats, worsens, or needs more support.
- **Closing reminder:** Before asking, *What is wrong with me?* ask, *What changed?*

References

Atherley, A., Dolmans, D., Hu, W., Hegazi, I., Alexander, S., & Teunissen, P. W. (2019). Beyond the struggles: A scoping review on the transition to undergraduate clinical training. *Medical Education, 53*(6), 559–570. doi:10.1111/medu.13883.

Butler, A. C. (2010). Repeated testing produces superior transfer of learning relative to repeated studying. *Journal of Experimental Psychology: Learning, Memory, and Cognition, 36*(5), 1118–1133. doi:10.1037/a0019902.

Dai, C. M., Bertram, K., & Chahine, S. (2021). Feedback credibility in healthcare education: A systematic review and synthesis. *Medical Science Educator, 31*(2), 923–933. doi:10.1007/s40670-020-01167-w.

Dornan, T., Boshuizen, H., King, N., & Scherpbier, A. (2007). Experience-based learning: A model linking the processes and outcomes of medical students' workplace learning. *Medical Education, 41*(1), 84–91. doi:10.1111/j.1365-2929.2006.02652.x.

Eva, K. W., & Regehr, G. (2005). Self-assessment in the health professions: A reformulation and research agenda. *Academic Medicine, 80*(10 Suppl), S46–S54. doi:10.1097/00001888-200510001-00015.

Eva, K. W., & Regehr, G. (2011). Exploring the divergence between self-assessment and self-monitoring. *Advances in Health Sciences Education, 16*(3), 311–329. doi:10.1007/s10459-010-9263-2.

Fuentes-Cimma, J., Sluijsmans, D., Riquelme, A., Villagran, I., Isbej, L., Olivares-Labbe, M. T., & Heeneman, S. (2024). Designing feedback processes in the workplace-based learning of undergraduate health professions education: A scoping review. *BMC Medical Education, 24*, 440. doi:10.1186/s12909-024-05439-6.

Gingerich, A., Kogan, J., Yeates, P., Govaerts, M., & Holmboe, E. (2014). Seeing the "black box" differently: Assessor cognition from three research perspectives. *Medical Education, 48*(11), 1055–1068. doi:10.1111/medu.12546.

Gottlieb, M., Chan, T. M., Zaver, F., & Ellaway, R. (2022). Confidence-competence alignment and the role of self-confidence in medical education: A conceptual review. *Medical Education, 56*(1), 37–47. doi:10.1111/medu.14592.

Hafferty, F. W., & Franks, R. (1994). The hidden curriculum, ethics teaching, and the structure of medical education. *Academic Medicine, 69*(11), 861–871. doi:10.1097/00001888-199411000-00001.

Han, P. K. J., Klein, W. M. P., & Arora, N. K. (2011). Varieties of uncertainty in health care: A conceptual taxonomy. *Medical Decision Making, 31*(6), 828–838. doi:10.1177/0272989X10393976.

Johnson, W. R., Durning, S. J., Allard, R. J., Barelski, A. M., & Artino, A. R., Jr. (2023). A scoping review of self-monitoring in graduate medical education. *Medical Education, 57*(9), 795–806. doi:10.1111/medu.15023.

Kennedy, T. J. T., Lingard, L., Baker, G. R., Kitchen, L., & Regehr, G. (2007). Clinical oversight: Conceptualizing the relationship between supervision and safety. *Journal of General Internal Medicine, 22*(8), 1080–1085. doi:10.1007/s11606-007-0179-3.

Kennedy, T. J. T., Regehr, G., Baker, G. R., & Lingard, L. (2009). Preserving professional credibility: Grounded theory study of medical trainees' requests for clinical support. *BMJ, 338*, b128. doi:10.1136/bmj.b128.

Larsen, D. P., Butler, A. C., & Roediger, H. L., III. (2008). Test-enhanced learning in medical education. *Medical Education, 42*(10), 959–966. doi:10.1111/j.1365-2923.2008.03124.x.

Lawrence, C., Mhlaba, T., Stewart, K. A., Moletsane, R., Gaede, B., & Moshabela, M. (2018). The hidden curricula of medical education: A scoping review. *Academic Medicine, 93*(4), 648–656. doi:10.1097/ACM.0000000000002004.

Lee, C., Hall, K., Anakin, M., & Pinnock, R. (2021). Towards a new understanding of uncertainty in medical education. *Journal of Evaluation in Clinical Practice, 27*(5), 1194–1204. doi:10.1111/jep.13503.

McClintock, A. H., Fainstad, T., Blau, K., & Jauregui, J. (2023). Psychological safety in medical education: A scoping review and synthesis of the literature. *Medical Teacher, 45*(11), 1290–1299. doi:10.1080/0142159X.2023.2216863.

McGaghie, W. C., Issenberg, S. B., Cohen, E. R., Barsuk, J. H., & Wayne, D. B. (2011). Does simulation-based medical education with deliberate practice yield better results than traditional clinical education? A meta-analytic comparative review of the evidence. *Academic Medicine, 86*(6), 706–711. doi:10.1097/ACM.0b013e318217e119.

Mylopoulos, M., & Regehr, G. (2009). How student models of expertise and innovation impact the development of adaptive expertise in medicine. *Medical Education, 43*(2), 127–132. doi:10.1111/j.1365-2923.2008.03254.x.

Mylopoulos, M., & Woods, N. N. (2017). When I say ... adaptive expertise. *Medical Education, 51*(7), 685–686. doi:10.1111/medu.13247.

Norman, G. (2005). Research in clinical reasoning: Past history and current trends. *Medical Education, 39*(4), 418–427. doi:10.1111/j.1365-2929.2005.02127.x.

Roediger, H. L., III, & Karpicke, J. D. (2006). Test-enhanced learning: Taking memory tests improves long-term retention. *Psychological Science, 17*(3), 249–255. doi:10.1111/j.1467-9280.2006.01693.x.

Sanderson, P., McCurdie, T., & Grundgeiger, T. (2019). Interruptions in health care: Assessing their connection with error and patient harm. *Human Factors, 61*(7), 1025–1036. doi:10.1177/0018720819869115.

Schmidt, H. G., & Rikers, R. M. J. P. (2007). How expertise develops in medicine: Knowledge encapsulation and illness script formation. *Medical Education, 41*(12), 1133–1139. doi:10.1111/j.1365-2923.2007.02915.x.

Schumacher, D. J., Michelson, C., Winn, A. S., Turner, D. A., Elshoff, E., & Kinnear, B. (2022). Making prospective entrustment decisions: Knowing limits, seeking help and defaulting. *Medical Education, 56*(9), 892–900. doi:10.1111/medu.14797.

Seoane, H. A., Moschetto, L., Orliacq, F., Orliacq, J., Serrano, E., Cazenave, M. I., Vigo, D. E., & Perez-Lloret, S. (2020). Sleep disruption in medicine students and its relationship with impaired academic performance: A systematic review and meta-analysis. *Sleep Medicine Reviews, 53*, 101333. doi:10.1016/j.smrv.2020.101333.

Telio, S., Ajjawi, R., & Regehr, G. (2015). The "educational alliance" as a framework for reconceptualizing feedback in medical education. *Academic Medicine, 90*(5), 609–614. doi:10.1097/ACM.0000000000000560.

Telio, S., Regehr, G., & Ajjawi, R. (2016). Feedback and the educational alliance: Examining credibility judgements and their consequences. *Medical Education, 50*(9), 933–942. doi:10.1111/medu.13063.

ten Cate, O. (2013). Nuts and bolts of entrustable professional activities. *Journal of Graduate Medical Education, 5*(1), 157–158. doi:10.4300/JGME-D-12-00380.1.

Teunissen, P. W., & Westerman, M. (2011). Opportunity or threat: The ambiguity of the consequences of transitions in medical education. *Medical Education, 45*(1), 51–59. doi:10.1111/j.1365-2923.2010.03755.x.

Watling, C., Driessen, E., van der Vleuten, C. P. M., & Lingard, L. (2012). Learning from clinical work: The roles of learning cues and credibility judgements. *Medical Education, 46*(2), 192–200. doi:10.1111/j.1365-2923.2011.04126.x.

Westbrook, J. I., Coiera, E., Dunsmuir, W. T. M., Brown, B. M., Kelk, N., Paoloni, R., & Tran, C. (2010). The impact of interruptions on clinical task completion. *Quality & Safety in Health Care, 19*(4), 284–289. doi:10.1136/qshc.2009.039255.

Yates, N., Gough, S., & Brazil, V. (2022). Self-assessment: With all its limitations, why are we still measuring and teaching it? Lessons from a scoping review. *Medical Teacher, 44*(11), 1296–1302. doi:10.1080/0142159X.2022.2093704.